Contents

Foreword: American inpatient psychiatry in historical perspective

In 1847, Horace Buttolph, one of the early members of the Association of Medical Superintendents of American Institutions for the Insane (AMSAII, now called the American Psychiatric Association, APA),[1] outlined the ideal treatment for individuals with the condition known at the time as insanity. Appropriate care for patients involved placement in a carefully designed building with a supportive environment and a trained staff. Buttolph emphasized that this atmosphere of care and support was dramatically different from that experienced by insane individuals in the past, who "were treated as outcasts from society, as alike unworthy of the care of friends, and the sympathy of their kind. By some, they were supposed to be possessed of evil spirits, and exorcism resorted to for their relief, by others, they were deemed sorcerers, and burned at the stake, without even a form of justice in their behalf" (p. 371 [1]). Buttolph encouraged national agreement on the humane care for the insane, "until the enlightened benevolence of modern times, has done all in its power to relieve the dark picture of their suffering and neglect, in the history of the past" (p. 378) [1]).

Many modern individuals (including some mental health professionals) now view nineteenth-century asylums as specters of the dark history of psychiatry. But at the time of its origin, the asylum was viewed as a revolutionary and beneficial institution. Indeed, for the first century after the founding of the APA, members celebrated the history of the asylum as the story of progress in the care of the mentally ill. Henry M. Hurd's *The Institutional Care of the Insane in the United States and Canada*, one of the first histories of American psychiatry, explored the origins of psychiatric hospitals across the nation and provided individual histories of all the nation's institutions [2]. In hindsight today, it might seem odd that the history of institutional psychiatry preceded that of psychoanalysis [3], but in fact the history of inpatient psychiatry is the history of psychiatry itself. Before hospitals became central locations for treatment of medical illnesses [4], psychiatric institutions served major social and public health functions in the United States.

---

[1] The Association of Medical Superintendents of American Institutions for the Insane was founded in 1844 and changed its name to the American Medico-Psychological Association in 1892. It became the American Psychiatric Association in 1920. The journal associated with the organization began in 1844 as the *American Journal of Insanity*, but became the *American Journal of Psychiatry* in 1920.

Much of the terminology has changed in the treatment of the mentally ill over the last two centuries. In the nineteenth century, it was common to talk about mental alienation or insanity rather than mental illness, while psychiatric hospitals were frequently called asylums or institutions for the insane. The reasons why patients would be identified as in need of treatment changed, as social and professional interpretations of individual behavior shifted [5]. Treatments have also changed, from moral therapy, to active somatic treatments such as hydrotherapy, convulsive therapies and lobotomy, to medications. Further, the focus of American psychiatry has shifted, from a nineteenth-century emphasis on institutional care through a mid-twentieth century move toward addressing the problems of neurotic outpatients, to the modern broad, encompassing view of psychiatric illness in the population. Yet throughout most of the last two centuries, psychiatric hospitals of some kind have been critical to the care of mentally ill individuals.

The history of inpatient psychiatry in the United States reminds us that we have always practiced at the nexus of patient difficulties, family concerns, state and federal policies, and broader social factors that affect our treatment of the mentally ill. Psychiatrists have always had to advocate for mentally ill patients and balance the benefits and drawbacks of psychiatric institutions. Today, at a time when teams of mental health workers in psychiatric hospitals are attempting to grapple with the fast pace, enormous demands, limited reimbursement, and complicated patient populations inherent in current inpatient psychiatry, it is important to reflect on how we got here. In the cycles of history, we have come around once more to a time when we need to advocate for inpatient psychiatry and to make the observation that this treatment setting requires special expertise.

1830s–1900: Moral therapy

Although the first few institutions to house the insane were opened in the eighteenth century, the impetus for states to build asylums for the insane came from reform movements in the middle of the nineteenth century [6]. One of the most vocal and active reformers in this time period, Dorothea Dix, traveled around the country and beseeched congressmen and community leaders to pay heed to the plight of the insane [7, 8]. Dix emphasized that these unfortunate individuals were often sequestered in prisons and poorhouses, or even left out on the streets to fend for themselves. Dix advocated for the construction of institutions for these individuals that would provide structure, security, and a healing environment. In her reform endeavors, Dix often partnered with members of a newly organized medical organization, the AMSAII (now the APA) [9].

Dix and the members of the AMSAII shared a conviction that the insane required appropriate institutions – asylums – to protect them from the harsh social and economic realities that contributed to (or caused) mental derangement [10]. At the time when Dix and others were active in reform efforts throughout the United States, institution building appeared to be the most progressive and humane measure to help people in need [11]. And Dix and her cohort of reformers succeeded in spurring state legislations to construct facilities for the insane across the country by the beginning of the twentieth century [2].

Historian Patricia D'Antonio has pointed out that the mid-nineteenth-century insane asylum was an institution based on negotiations between family and emerging psychiatric ideals and practices. Encounters among patients, staff, and families were not incidental parts of the treatment but rather these interactions constituted treatment within the therapeutic environment [12]. As historian Nancy Tomes has masterfully illustrated, the idea behind mental institutions in the nineteenth century was that patients experienced a moral environment – characterized by healthy staff relationships, good food, pleasant surroundings, and productive activities – in order to resolve their insanity. Most nineteenth-century asylums were modeled on the example set by Pennsylvania psychiatrist Thomas Kirkbride at the Pennsylvania Hospital for the Insane, where the physical architecture and internal organization influenced generations of psychiatrists. At the head of an institution on the Kirkbride model was the superintendent who acted as a father figure. His staff, including the heads of the male and female departments, were also members of the family and helped to govern. The atmosphere of culture and civility was intended to illustrate to the patients the appropriate way to behave in society. Presumably the example they experienced while in the asylum would help them become adjusted to life outside [13].

It is remarkable from our distance in time to reflect on public attitudes toward insane asylums in the nineteenth century. Although we might think of patients locked away and forgotten, the reality appears to have been quite different for many. As Tomes has described, patients within Kirkbride's asylum often accepted and appreciated the care they were provided. They understood their role within the institution, and wrote to Kirkbride to seek advice even after discharge. Kirkbride's associates with the AMSAII shared the expectation that their services and their role within the institution would be valued by the patients, and patients often fulfilled that expectation. In 1849, for example, members of the AMSAII toured several local mental institutions in New York in the course of their annual meeting. At the New York State Lunatic Asylum, a patient (and former minister) spoke for an assembly of more than 300 patients to express gratitude and support for the visiting members of the association: "The presence of a voluntary association of medical gentlemen devoted to the noblest branch of the healing art, the care and recovery of the diseased mind, is calculated to awaken sentiments of gratitude and respect. And for myself and fellow patients, I would greet you with a respectful and cordial welcome. . .our duty to that unfortunate class of our fellow citizens who are afflicted with insanity, seems to demand that they should not only have the benefit of all that wealth can furnish for their comfort but also of the highest medical wisdom and skill which those can secure to whose care they are committed by their friends as an important trust" (pp. 12–13 [14]). Certainly at least some patients were able to understand and appreciate that they were experiencing the best that American psychiatry had to offer at the time.

But not all patients in the nineteenth century were able to receive care from national leaders in psychiatry or stay in well appointed asylums. Historian Ellen Dwyer compared the care of patients in two nineteenth-century asylums and found that patients experienced radically different courses of illness and treatment. Although psychiatrist leaders in the best institutions likened their asylums to large families, patients in less elite locations might have experienced their stay as more like a prison sentence. While some institutions took care of patients who were more acutely ill and attempted to discharge them within weeks to months, other facilities took on chronic cases in which the hospital stay might last for years to decades [15]. As historian Gerald Grob has observed, overcrowding and increasing numbers of chronic cases made the reality of asylum life much less than the ideal in some institutions [6].

Not only were experiences different based on patient class and illness course, but also race and region played a large role in institutional psychiatry in the nineteenth century. As Peter McCandless has described, the history of the care of the insane in South Carolina illustrates the broad disparities in asylum experiences due to race and social structure. Before the Civil War, few black patients were admitted to the South Carolina asylum as their behavior was effectively controlled within the institution of slavery, while most white insane individuals had sufficient community support to avoid institutions. After the war, however, South Carolina experienced a rapid decline in economic power as a whole, and insane individuals were less likely to be cared for by their families. In addition, the state asylum began to accept black patients in segregated, inferior wards. In this environment, it was hard to believe that the environment was therapeutic for anyone, especially black patients [16].

Though nineteenth-century patients and psychiatrists generally shared a conviction that institutions were helpful and humane, the profession by the early twentieth century began to shift their attention away from the asylum. Many psychiatrists by the turn of the century experienced loss of control over their institutions as state mental health offices began to dictate policy [17]. Also, as historian Elizabeth Lunbeck has described, some in the profession began to look beyond the confines of psychiatric institutions to promote psychiatric expertise throughout society [18]. In addition, psychiatrists became increasingly aware that the institution itself – especially the detail around building maintenance – was drawing criticism from other medical professions, including psychiatrists' closest professional competitors, neurologists [19, 20]. Critics – including neurologist S. Weir Mitchell who addressed the professional association's meeting in 1894 – accused American psychiatrists of being more interested in the maintenance of their buildings than the care of their patients [21]. It was not enough to put patients in grand institutions and expect them to get better. Psychiatrists needed to do more for the patients.

1900s–1960s: Treatment in the hospital

By the early twentieth century, the promise of psychiatric cure through institutional care was beginning to dim. The numbers and types of institutions were growing at a high rate and some kinds of individuals appeared relegated to custodial care rather than treatment [22]. In a few locations, research-minded psychiatrists created new kinds of institutions, psychopathic hospitals, to permit shorter hospital stays and promote research and active treatment. But though these hospitals – including the State Psychopathic Hospital at the University of Michigan, the Boston Psychopathic Hospital, the New York State Psychiatric Institute, and the Henry Phipps Clinic at the Johns Hopkins University – were influential, they did not provide the bulk of psychiatric care to patients in the twentieth century [18, 23, 24]. Instead, the major change during this time period was that large psychiatric institutions, now mostly public and private mental hospitals, tried to meet the challenges of care for increasing numbers of patients at the same time that they seized opportunities for treatment innovation [25].

As historian and psychiatrist Joel Braslow has described, in the first half of the twentieth century American psychiatrists used somatic therapies on hospitalized psychiatric patients, including hydrotherapy, malarial fever therapy, sexual sterilization, and convulsive therapy [26]. Hydrotherapy, which originated in the nineteenth century, involved immersing patients in large tubs of water and/or wrapping them in wet sheets. Malarial fever therapy (in which patients were inoculated with serum from patients with active malaria) was used to treat patients with tertiary syphilis after it was observed that the high fevers in patients with malaria appeared to kill the organism responsible for syphilis. Sexual sterilization, most often performed in women, was intended to remove the sexual urges that psychiatrists believed fueled some psychoses [27]. All of these treatments, including convulsive therapy – one form of which is in use today – were intended to tackle the obvious and troubling problem of severe agitation in hospitalized patients. These interventions appeared to be helpful, scientific, and offered the promise of genuine treatment of cases that previously appeared hopeless.

Practitioners (as well as the public) were especially enthusiastic about convulsive therapy, including insulin coma therapy, metrazol therapy, and electroconvulsive therapy (ECT). Insulin coma therapy, which came about after the discovery of insulin in the 1920s [28], involved having patients receive increasing doses of insulin to the point that they went into a coma and/or experienced convulsions before they were revived with a sugar solution. By the 1930s, psychiatrists who worked with this technique proclaimed major benefit to severely ill patients, especially those with schizophrenia [29]. Other theorists and practitioners developed alternative ways of producing convulsions, which also seemed to help patients, including use of the drug metrazol in which individuals with manic depressive psychoses and involutional melancholia appeared to respond best [30].

Of course, the most well known physical intervention to be developed and used in the context of psychiatric institutions was ECT. Although ECT originated in Italy in the 1930s, ECT techniques and practitioners spread rapidly throughout the world by the 1940s [31]. Electroconvulsive therapy enthusiasts were aware of the potential dangers of ECT (which at the time of its introduction included fractures as anesthesia was not routinely given until the 1960s), but the treatment offered hope for patients who were so ill that they could not leave psychiatric hospitals. Although we now tend to think of ECT and psychotherapy as almost completely opposite, practitioners in the 1940s and 1950s imagined a more fluid relationship among the treatment modalities. For example, at the time when psychoanalytic concepts became more prevalent within American psychiatry [32], many interpreted the action of ECT in psychodynamic terms [33].

Somatic therapies flourished in psychiatric hospitals in the first half of the twentieth century partly because psychiatrists were desperate to be doing something to help their patients. As conditions worsened in the hospitals, some psychiatrists became even more aggressive with their interventions. By the 1940s, increasing numbers of chronic and older patients made overcrowding in hospitals worse [34]. Further, journalistic exposés of hospital environments created public awareness and pressure on hospital physicians to take action [35]. As historian Jack Pressman pointed out, hospital overcrowding, deteriorating hospital conditions, and poor prognosis of patients led to increasing professional and public enthusiasm for heroic therapies – including frontal lobotomy. Although we now view the history of lobotomy as a dark episode in psychiatry's past [36], Pressman explained that many psychiatrists in the 1940s saw the introduction of psychosurgery as a promising development [37]. Indeed, lobotomy and shock therapies were concrete, physical therapies that could be measured, they addressed the severity of the problems of the mentally ill in institutions, and they appeared to represent application of scientific thinking to psychiatric problems. For practitioners and researchers who used the efficacy standards of the time [38], these somatic therapies worked.

Although most of the somatic treatments developed in twentieth-century institutions did not last in psychiatrists' therapeutic repertoire, the hospital setting provided the impetus for our most lasting intervention – psychiatric medications. While institutionally based psychiatrists were not shy about using ECT and/or lobotomy for seriously ill patients, these interventions did not succeed in managing all patients. In the years after World War II and the worldwide success of penicillin, pharmaceutical companies began to look to expand their medication offerings [39]. Psychiatric hospitals appeared to be an ideal location in which to test new pharmaceutical agents – the populations were large, the existing treatments had not removed the problem of the seriously ill, and it was easy (in the days before informed consent and Institutional Review Boards [IRBs]) [40] to give medications to patients to see what would happen [41, 42].

Medication development in psychiatric hospitals not only led to the introduction of major classes of drugs (beginning with chlorpromazine and imipramine), but also helped to classify psychiatric patients. Through medication trials in the 1960s and 1970s, patients who responded to the different drugs were grouped into separate diagnostic categories [43, 44]. Their symptoms were then counted and listed, which led to the symptom-based diagnoses in the watershed third edition of the *Diagnostic and Statistical Manual* (DSM-III) in 1980 [45]. As Joel Braslow and Sarah Starks have further described, the introduction of psychiatric medications to hospitalized patient populations also expanded the number and type of patients who were potentially helped by psychiatric interventions, including those with everyday problems of living [46].

The introduction of medications, as well as the shift of many older patients out of psychiatric hospitals and into nursing homes, helped lead to the decline of psychiatric institutions as the major centers for psychiatric care [47]. For the first time, large numbers of patients were discharged from the hospitals and many returned to their communities. Further, social and cultural changes in the United States helped to translate the older criticism of overcrowded institutions into a widespread critique of psychiatric hospitals in general. Since the 1960s, psychiatric hospitals have been the target of widespread hostility, and their past was condemned as well as their present.

1960s–1980s: Community care

In 1963, President John F. Kennedy signed the Community Mental Health Centers Act, which formalized the shift in mental health policy priority from institutions to outpatient care. Yet as historian Gerald Grob has pointed out, community mental health centers could more easily deal with neurotic outpatients than the seriously mentally ill patients who had been in hospitals. In the 1960s, hospitals began to transfer patients out of the hospital and into communities that did not have the resources to handle them [48, 49]. Not only were the communities not set up for the sickest patients, but also there were fewer providers willing to take on their care. By this time period, more psychiatrists had become entranced by the possibilities of psychoanalysis and outpatient practice [32, 47]. The flood of both patients and practitioners away from institutional settings led to major social problems. By the 1970s and 1980s, especially in places such as New York City and Los Angeles, it was clear that many patients were failing to make an effective transition from institutional care to community living [50]. Indeed, the flow of patients back onto the streets and into the jails was reminiscent of the social plight that Dorothea Dix had attempted to address more than a century earlier [51].

But there was nothing inevitable about the problems that resulted from the deinstitutionalization movement, and in fact the abandonment of the hospital as part of the transition toward community care was not necessary. As historian John Burnham has pointed out with the example of the mental health system in Topeka, KS, it was possible for the community mental health center and hospital to partner in the process of getting patients help and support across the spectrum of care [52]. But though the continuity between hospital and community worked in Topeka (perhaps because of the influence of the Menninger family) [53], the Topeka model was not widely emulated in the United States due to widespread rejection of state psychiatric hospitals and a widening conflict between state and federal mental health policy [54].

Indeed, psychiatric institutions appeared so problematic to critics and social commentators by the 1970s that even their histories were rife with criticism. Theorists such as Michel Foucault in France and David Rothman and Andrew Scull in the United States described the history of psychiatric hospitals as the history of state-sanctioned repressive and dictatorial practices directed at vulnerable individuals [55, 56, 57]. Antagonism toward mental hospitals was taken up by growing numbers of individuals who protested psychiatry in general [58]. Emerging patients' rights groups also strongly suggested that psychiatric hospitals did not help the mentally ill, and some argued that hospitals were more like prisons than healing institutions [59, 60].

For those hospitals that did remain, the environment inside and outside the institution became contentious. As patients demanded rights within psychiatric hospitals, changes in commitment laws formalized civil proceedings for patients who appeared to be mentally ill and in need of treatment [61]. Further, hospital beds funded by states significantly declined while beds within private hospitals increased [62]. Although mentally ill individuals still required periodic hospitalization, these episodes of care were not discussed often within national professional venues. Leaders of the psychiatric profession focused on increasingly complex issues such as federal support for mental health research, while others emphasized psychiatric diagnostic systems and development of further medications for mental illness [63, 64]. Few in organized psychiatry were taking up the issue of hospital care as the number of available psychiatric hospital beds continued to shrink across the country.

During the decades of state and national focus on outpatient mental health care, psychiatric hospitals were seldom discussed and were not incorporated into policy discussions around the mentally ill. But even as many in the profession had little or no interest in institutional care, small groups of psychiatrists continued to insist that psychiatric hospitals could play an important role, and that special interventions and techniques were necessary in this setting [65, 66]. Early in the twentieth century, psychiatric institutions had begun to actively employ staff such as social workers and activity therapists in order to enhance patients' experiences in the hospital [67]. By the 1960s and 1970s, hospital-based psychiatrists were emphasizing the importance of inter-disciplinary work and the combination of somatic, group, and psychotherapy techniques they found ideal in this setting [68]. By the 1970s and 1980s, as state psychiatric hospitals continued to close and move their patients into the community, psychiatric units of general hospitals became increasingly important to mental health care [69]. In addition, health service researchers pointed out that the remaining state facilities were serving some purpose in the broad context of psychiatric care [70]. Although many psychiatric hospitals by this time period employed private practice models (in which private practitioners had admitting privileges to inpatient units), some dedicated psychiatric staffs and academic centers worked to develop a consistent hospital environment for the patients who passed through the revolving door [71].

Reinvigorated inpatient psychiatry

At the same time that psychiatric hospitals' role decreased in the care of the mentally ill, the role of the general medical hospital changed as well. Although technological changes and advances in treatment expanded, the rising costs of hospital care and the influence of third-party payment decreased hospital lengths of stay [72]. As a result, the patients in general hospitals over the last 20 years have been increasingly sick with more and more rapid turnover. In this context, it has become evident to many medical specialties that patients in the hospital require a more intense level of care and greater expertise [73]. A group of general physicians founded the National Association of Inpatient Physicians in 1998 (the organization changed its name to the Society of Hospital Medicine in 2003) in order to address the increasing acuity of hospitalized patients [74]. In the last decade, the concept of the hospitalist – a physician who specializes in the hospital treatment of the ill – has become much more common in general medical care.

In psychiatry, too, a small but growing number of psychiatrists have begun to reclaim hospital-based psychiatry with the same model as the general hospital specialist [75]. Modern-day hospitalists have also emphasized the importance – perhaps even the centrality – of the acute care psychiatric hospital to the mentally ill. Further, hospitalist models are increasingly dominating residency training [76]. As has been clear for more than a century, psychiatric institutions provide potentially ideal places to engage in meaning-ful research to develop new and more effective treatments. Further, the inten-sive nature of inpatient care allows for engagement with patients on a different level than the more sporadic contacts in outpatient care. But with the reinvigoration of hospital psychiatry, current practitioners inherit the long history of American psychiatry as a whole and continue to face opportunities as well as challenges in this work.

Although many of the challenges inherent in inpatient psychiatric care are not new, they remain important and require ongoing attention on a personal and a policy level. First, gender, race, and class continue to affect patients' hospital care experiences, despite well intentioned physicians and staff. All major psychiatric treatment innovations, from ECT to lobotomy to medications, have been given more often to women than to men in psychiatric hospitals [26, 37, 46, 77], while men formed the bulk of the patient group treated for alcohol and drug problems [78]. In addition, the ways in which physicians have traditionally understood and treated patients based on race have skewed their interpretations of normality and disease [79, 80]. As Stephen Jay Gould reminded us, it is important to understand the ways in which our culture and society frame our expectations about individuals and the interventions they appear to need [81].

Not only do gender and race considerations need to be part of careful inpatient psychiatric care, but also research opportunities can blind us to the risks of investigating acute and high-risk patient populations. History reminds us that it is important to remain humble and not to expect that one radical solution exists for the problem of mental illness [82]. As the history of lobotomy illustrates, a sincere desire to help seriously ill patients can lead to drastic interventions without adequate checks and balances [37]. Even now, as David Healy has pointed out, there is significant potential for psychiatrists to become too enamored of the power and influence associated with the pharmaceutical industry and its sponsorship of research without adequate concerns for the patients who might experience harm from recklessly marketed drugs [83].

Finally, inpatient psychiatry in the twenty-first century involves layers of challenges unimaginable to psychiatrists from more than a century ago. While psychiatric hospital leaders in the early twentieth century pioneered in tabulating patient data and gathering statistics, they could not possibly have foreseen the quantity and diverse audiences of modern documentation requirements. Further, while hospitals in the past struggled with finances and the balance between paying and charity patients [6], our current mix of public and private insurers has led to a maddening maze of reimbursement policies that encapsulate the conflict between insurers' desire to pay as little as possible and hospitals' efforts to maximize payments [84]. While our nineteenth-century predecessors complained about having to answer to the authority of state governments, hospital boards, and professional organizations, they did not have the multitude of involved groups peering over their shoulders the way that current hospital psychiatrists experience. Even as our methods for managing information have evolved, so have our obligations to share information with different parties expanded.

Early twentieth-century Harvard philosopher George Santayana made a now well known comment about the value of remembering history. It is worth looking at the few sentences preceding his famous comment: "Progress, far from consisting in change, depends on retentiveness. When change is absolute there remains no being to improve and no direction is set for possible improvement: and when experience is not retained, as among savages, infancy is perpetual. Those who cannot remember the past are condemned to repeat it" (p. 284 [85]). As we reinvent inpatient psychiatry for a new generation, it is essential that we remember what has gone before. We need our history – good, bad, and indifferent – in order to continue to grow. Modern psychiatric hospital physicians are engaged in the most traditional work in the history of psychiatry – the care of seriously ill patients within institutions. Like our predecessors more than a century ago, the ability to take care of these patients requires special skills and a comprehensive awareness of psychopathology and tools to manage behavior. As Michael Casher and Joshua Bess illustrate in this book, inpatient psychiatry remains an exciting challenge to modern practitioners at the historically most important site of care: the hospital.

Further reading

In addition to the citations already provided, interested readers should avail themselves of two outstanding surveys of the history of American psychiatry. Edward Shorter completed an account of psychiatry's transformation over the last century and a half, focusing on somatic treatments and comparisons with Europe [86]. Historian Gerald Grob, one of the most well respected experts in the history of psychiatry, completed not only a three-volume exploration of American psychiatry (cited in several places above), but also wrote a one-volume overview that is accessible, informative, and provides an ideal introduction to the history of psychiatry [87].

The history of institutional psychiatric care in countries outside the United States is broad and complex. The most prolific author on the topic of British and international psychiatry was the late Roy Porter, whose voluminous works covered the history of madness, the history of British institutions, and surveys of international institutional psychiatry [88, 89, 90].

Laura D. Hirshbein

References

1. Buttolph H A. Modern asylums. *American Journal of Insanity*, **3** (1847), 364–78.

2. Hurd H M ed. *The Institutional Care of the Insane in the United States and Canada.* Baltimore: Johns Hopkins Press; 1916.

3. Micale M S & Porter R eds. *Discovering the History of Psychiatry.* New York: Oxford University Press; 1994.

4. Rosenberg C E. *The Care of Strangers: The Rise of America's Hospital System.* New York: Basic Books; 1987.

5. Fox R W. *So Far Disordered in Mind: Insanity in California, 1870–1930*. Berkeley: University of California Press; 1978.

6. Grob G N. *Mental Institutions in America: Social Policy to 1875*. New York: Free Press; 1973.

7. Gollaher D L. *Voice for the Mad: The Life of Dorothea Dix*. New York: Free Press; 1995.

8. Brown T J. *Dorothea Dix: New England Reformer*. Cambridge: Harvard University Press; 1998.

9. Barton W E. *The History and Influence of the American Psychiatric Association*. Washington, DC: American Psychiatric Press; 1987.

10. McGovern C M. *Masters of Madness: Social Origins of the American Psychiatric Profession*. Hanover, NH: University Press of New England; 1985.

11. Walters R G. *American Reformers, 1815–1860*. New York: Hill and Wang; 1978.

12. D'Antonio P. *Founding Friends: Families, Staff, and Patients at the Friends Asylum in Early Nineteenth-Century Philadelphia*. Bethlehem, PA: Lehigh University Press; 2006.

13. Tomes N. *The Art of Asylum-Keeping: Thomas Story Kirkbride and the Origins of American Psychiatry*. Philadelphia, PA: University of Pennsylvania Press; 1994.

14. Fourth Annual Meeting of the Association for Medical Superintendents of American Institutions for the Insane. *American Journal of Insanity*, **6** (1849), 52–70.

15. Dwyer E. *Homes for the Mad: Life Inside Two Nineteenth-Century Asylums*. New Brunswick, NJ: Rutgers University Press; 1987.

16. McCandless P. *Moonlight, Magnolias, and Madness: Insanity in South Carolina From the Colonial Period to the Progressive Era*. Chapel Hill, NC: University of North Carolina Press; 1996.

17. Dowbiggin I. "Midnight clerks and daily drudges": hospital psychiatry in New York state, 1890–1905. *Journal of the History of Medicine and Allied Sciences*, **47** (1992), 130–52.

18. Lunbeck E. *The Psychiatric Persuasion: Knowledge, Gender, and Power in Modern America*. Princeton, NJ: Princeton University Press; 1994.

19. Rosenberg C E. *The Trial of the Assassin Guiteau: Psychiatry and Law in the Gilded Age*. Chicago, IL: University of Chicago Press; 1968.

20. Blustein B E. New York neurologists and the specialization of American medicine. *Bulletin of the History of Medicine*, **53** (1979), 170–83.

21. Mitchell S W. Address Before the Fiftieth Annual Meeting of the American Medico-Psychological Association: Philadelphia, May 16th, 1894. *Journal of Nervous & Mental Disease*, **21** (1894), 413–37.

22. Noll S. *Feeble-Minded in Our Midst: Institutions for the Mentally Retarded in the South, 1900–1940*. Chapel Hill, NC: University of North Carolina Press; 1995.

23. Kolb L C & Roizin L. *The First Psychiatric Institute: How Research and Education Changed Practice.* Washington, DC: American Psychiatric Press, Inc.; 1993.

24. Lidz T & Marx O. Adolph Meyer and psychiatric training at the Phipps Clinic: an interview with Theodore Lidz. *History of Psychiatry*, **4** (1993), 245–69.

25. Pols H. Divergences in American Psychiatry during the depression: somatic psychiatry, community mental hygiene, and social reconstruction. *Journal of the History of the Behavioral Sciences*, **37** (2001), 369–88.

26. Braslow J T. *Mental Ills and Bodily Cures: Psychiatric Treatment in the First Half of the Twentieth Century.* Berkeley, CA: University of California Press; 1997.

27. Braslow J T. In the name of therapeutics: the practice of sterilization in a California state hospital. *Journal of the History of Medicine & Allied Sciences*, **51** (1996), 29–51.

28. Bliss M. *The Discovery of Insulin.* Chicago, IL: University of Chicago Press; 1984.

29. Doroshow D B. Performing a cure for schizophrenia: insulin coma therapy on the wards. *Journal of the History of Medicine & Allied Sciences*, **62** (2007), 213–43.

30. McCrae N. "A violent thunderstorm": cardiazol treatment in British mental hospitals. *History of Psychiatry*, **17** (2006), 67–90.

31. Shorter E & Healy D. *Shock Therapy: A History of Electroconvulsive Treatment in Mental Illness.* New Brunswick, NJ: Rutgers University Press; 2007.

32. Hale N G, Jr. *The Rise and Crisis of Psychoanalysis in the United States: Freud and the Americans, 1917–1985.* New York: Oxford University Press; 1995.

33. Sadowsky J H. Beyond the metaphor of the pendulum: electroconvulsive therapy, psychoanalysis, and the styles of American psychiatry. *Journal of the History of Medicine & Allied Sciences*, **61** (2006), 1–25.

34. Grob G N. *Mental Illness and American Society, 1875–1940.* Princeton, NJ: Princeton University Press; 1983.

35. Deutsch A. *The Shame of the States.* New York: Harcourt Brace; 1948.

36. Valenstein E S. *Great and Desperate Cures: The Rise and Decline of Psychosurgery and Other Radical Treatments for Mental Illness.* New York: Basic Books; 1986.

37. Pressman J D. *Last Resort: Psychosurgery and the Limits of Medicine.* New York: Cambridge University Press; 1998.

38. Marks H M. *The Progress of Experiment: Science and Therapeutic Reform in the United States, 1900–1990.* New York: Cambridge University Press; 1997.

39. Temin P. *Taking Your Medicine: Drug Regulation in the United States.* Cambridge, MA: Harvard University Press; 1980.

40. Lederer S E. *Subjected to Science: Human Experimentation in America Before the Second World War.* Baltimore, MD: Johns Hopkins University Press; 1995.

41. Healy D. *The Creation of Psychopharmacology.* Cambridge, MA: Harvard University Press; 2002.

42. Starks S L & Braslow J T. The making of contemporary American psychiatry, Part 1: Patients, treatments, and therapeutic rationales. *History of Psychology*, **8** (2005), 176–93.

43. Healy D. *The Antidepressant Era*. Cambridge, MA: Harvard University Press; 1997.

44. Hirshbein L D. *American Melancholy: Constructions of Depression in the Twentieth Century*. New Brunswick, NJ: Rutgers University Press; 2009.

45. Kutchins H & Kirk S A. *Making Us Crazy: DSM, The Psychiatric Bible and the Creation of Mental Disorders*. New York: Free Press; 1997.

46. Braslow J T & Starks S L. The making of contemporary American psychiatry, Part 2: Therapeutics and gender before and after World War II. *History of Psychology*, **8** (2005), 271–88.

47. Grob G N. *From Asylum to Community: Mental Health Policy in Modern America*. Princeton, NJ: Princeton University Press; 1991.

48. Grob G N. The paradox of deinstitutionalization. *Society*, **32** (1995), 51–9.

49. Grob G N. The severely and chronically mentally ill in America: retrospect and prospect. In: Leavitt J. W. & Numbers R. L. eds., *Sickness and Health in America.* Madison, WI: University of Wisconsin Press; 1997, pp. 334–48.

50. Bennett M I, Gudeman J E, Jenkins L, Brown A & Bennett M B. The value of hospital-based treatment for the homeless mentally ill. *American Journal of Psychiatry*, **145** (1988), 1273–6.

51. Morrissey J P & Goldman H H. Care and treatment of the mentally ill in the United States: historical developments and reforms. *Annals of the American Academy of Political and Social Science*, **1986** (484) (1986), 12–27.

52. Burnham J C. A clinical alternative to the public health approach to mental illness. *Perspectives in Biology and Medicine*, **49** (2006), 220–37.

53. Friedman L J. *Menninger: The Family and the Clinic*. New York: Knopf; 1990.

54. Grob G N & Goldman H H. *The Dilemma of Federal Mental Health Policy: Radical Reform or Incremental Change?* New Brunswick, NJ: Rutgers University Press; 2006.

55. Foucault M. *Madness and Civilization: A History of Insanity in the Age of Reason.* New York: Pantheon; 1967.

56. Rothman D J. *The Discovery of the Asylum: Social Order and Disorder in the New Republic.* Revised edn. Boston: Little, Brown and Company; 1990.

57. Scull A. *Social Order/Mental Disorder: Anglo-American Psychiatry in Historical Perspective*. Berkeley, CA: University of California Press; 1989.

58. Dain N. Critics and dissenters: reflections on "anti-psychiatry" in the United States. *Journal of the History of the Behavioral Sciences*, **25** (1989), 3–25.

59. Tomes N. The patient as a policy factor: a historical case study of the consumer/survivor movement in mental health. *Health Affairs*, **25** (2006), 720–9.

60. Beard P R. The consumer movement. In: Menninger R. W. & Nemiah J. C. eds., *American Psychiatry After World War II (1944–1994)*. Washington, DC: American Psychiatric Press; **2000**, pp. 299–320.

61. Appelbaum P S. *Almost a Revolution: Mental Health Law and the Limits of Change.* New York: Oxford University Press; 1994.

62. Dorwart R A, Schlesinger M, Davidson H, Epstein S & Hoover C. A national study of psychiatric hospital care. *American Journal of Psychiatry*, **148** (1991), 204–10.

63. Spiegel J P. Presidential address: Psychiatry – a high risk profession. *American Journal of Psychiatry*, **132** (1975), 693–7.

64. Gibson R W. Presidential address: A profession worthy of the public trust. *American Journal of Psychiatry*, **134** (1977), 723–8.

65. Lion J R, Adler W N, Webb W L, Jr, eds. *Modern Hospital Psychiatry*. New York: W. W. Norton & Company; 1988.

66. Taylor M A, Sierles F S & Abrams R, eds. *General Hospital Psychiatry.* New York: Free Press; 1985.

67. Quen J M. Asylum psychiatry, neurology, social work, and mental hygiene: an exploratory study in interprofessional history. *Journal of the History of the Behavioral Sciences*, **13** (1977), 3–11.

68. Abroms G M & Greenfield N S, eds. *The New Hospital Psychiatry.* New York: Academic Press; 1971.

69. Bachrach L L. General hospital psychiatry: overview from a sociological perspective. *American Journal of Psychiatry*, **138** (1981), 879–87.

70. Goldman H H, Taube C A, Regier D A & Witkin M. The multiple functions of the state mental hospital. *American Journal of Psychiatry*, **140** (1983), 296–300.

71. Fenton W S, Leaf P J, Moran N L & Tischler G L. Trends in psychiatric practice, 1965–1980. *American Journal of Psychiatry*, **141** (1984), 346–51.

72. Stevens R. In *Sickness and in Wealth: American Hospitals in the Twentieth Century.* New York: Basic Books; 1989.

73. Wachter R M & Goldman L. The emerging role of "hospitalists" in the American health care system. *New England Journal of Medicine*, **335** (1996), 514–17.

74. Wachter R M. Reflections: the hospitalist movement a decade later. *Journal of Hospital Medicine*, **1** (2006), 248–52.

75. Jerrard J. Psychiatric hospitalists diagnose, treat mental illness. *The Hospitalist*, October 2007.

76. Rabjohn P A & Yager J. The effects of resident work-hour regulation on psychiatry. *American Journal of Psychiatry*, **165** (2008), 308–11.

77. Hirshbein L D. Science, gender, and the emergence of depression in American psychiatry, 1952–1980. *Journal of the History of Medicine & Allied Sciences*, **61** (2006), 187–216.

78. Tracy S W. *Alcoholism in America: From Reconstruction to Prohibition*. Baltimore, MD: Johns Hopkins University Press; 2005.

79. Gambino M. "These strangers within our gates": race, psychiatry and mental illness among black Americans at St Elizabeth's Hospital in Washington, DC, 1900–40. *History of Psychiatry*, **19** (2008), 387–408.

80. Dwyer E. Psychiatry and race during World War II. *Journal of the History of Medicine & Allied Sciences*, **61** (2006), 117–43.

81. Gould S J. *The Mismeasure of Man*. Revised edn. New York: W. W. Norton & Company; 1996.

82. Scull A. *Madhouse: A Tragic Tale of Megalomania and Modern Medicine*. New Haven, CT: Yale University Press; 2005.

83. Healy D. *Let Them Eat Prozac: The Unhealthy Relationship Between the Pharmaceutical Industry and Depression*. New York: New York University Press; 2004.

84. Liptzin B, Gottlieb G L & Summergrad P. The future of psychiatric services in general hospitals. *American Journal of Psychiatry*, **164** (2007), 1468–72.

85. Santayana G. *The Life of Reason: The Phases of Human Progress*. Vol. I. New York: C. Scribner's Sons; 1905.

86. Shorter E. *A History of Psychiatry: From the Era of the Asylum to the Age of Prozac*. New York: John Wiley & Sons; 1997.

87. Grob G N. *The Mad Among Us: A History of the Care of America's Mentally Ill*. Cambridge, MA: Harvard University Press; 1994.

88. Porter R. *Madness: A Brief History*. New York: Oxford University Press; 2002.

89. Porter R & Wright D, eds., *The Confinement of the Insane: International Perspectives, 1800–1965*. New York: Cambridge University Press; 2003.

90. Porter R. Madness and its institutions. In: Wear A., ed. *Medicine in Society*. New York: Cambridge University Press; 1992, pp. 277–301.

Preface

Psychiatric units are the sites of lodging and treatment for many of the most challenging patients, including those with acute forms of serious Axis I disorders and regressed states of severe personality disorders. Inpatient psychiatry is a specialized area of psychiatric theory and practice that pertains to these hospital patients. It has many links with consultation psychiatry and emergency psychiatry. Clinicians in all three areas cope on a daily basis with the treatment challenges of patients with complex mixtures of mood and thought disorders, Axis II overlay, substance use, and medical illness.

Complicating inpatient psychiatric care even further are oft-found psychological issues of many patients, legal dilemmas of involuntary hospitalization, and extensive documentation requirements. In fact, consideration of the wide-reaching competencies essential to taking care of hospitalized psychiatric patients has led to increasing utilization of psychiatrist "hospitalists," a trend that parallels the directive in departments of internal medicine and neurology in many hospitals.

In this manual we offer an overview of the management of psychiatric inpatients, organized mostly according to the common diagnostic groupings found on an inpatient unit. No brief review can prepare inpatient practitioners for all the various circumstances they may encounter. That is certainly not our intent. There is no substitute for a firm grounding in the basic sciences of psychiatry, including psychopharmacology, psychiatric classification and differential diagnosis, psychology and psychodynamics (including family and group dynamics), and the related areas within medicine, including neurology and internal medicine. But our hope is that this streamlined synopsis can outline a majority of the main issues psychiatric practitioners will encounter on an inpatient unit, and help guide them in the daily care of patients.

In assembling this manual, in addition to reviewing the pertinent literature, we interviewed seasoned fellow psychiatrists. These trusted colleagues have demonstrated clinical know-how in the treatment of the types of patients most commonly presenting to hospital psychiatric units. Our collegial conversations fit well with the question/answer format of the book itself, in which we have tried to anticipate the kinds of general questions clinicians would have as they navigate the care of psychiatric inpatients. Readers will also find that our own personal philosophies of treatment are woven into the content of the manual, both explicitly – in boxes containing "pearls" from our own experience – but also by the emphasis throughout the book on sound clinical observation, flexibility of approach, and thorough consideration of treatment options.

This manual is designed to be of use to any and all inpatient clinicians and to assist them toward a sense of mastery in dealing with patients with psychotic illnesses, mood disorders, and personality disorders (especially borderline personality disorder, with its disproportionate presentation on the psychiatric unit). These days, with the United States and other countries awash with illicit drugs and abused prescription medications, and with the huge numbers of patients who cannot drink in moderation, it is also important that we have a firm grasp of the management of alcohol and chemical dependence and dual-diagnosis disorders. Because geriatric patients are also found on inpatient units, and are often referred for stabilization of dementia-related agitation, we have included a section on dementia-related psychiatric disorders. Also incorporated is a section on traumatic brain injury, which is increasingly recognized as associated with psychiatric disturbance, and treatment of which demands an integration of neurology, psychiatry, and physical medicine and rehabilitation. Rounding out the manual are two chapters that are not diagnosis focused but which address two areas that are of interest and concern in doing inpatient psychiatry. One chapter is a review of the issues involved in caring for the young adult on an inpatient psychiatric unit, and the other is a chapter devoted to the quotidian, yet essential, issue of psychiatric documentation.

Acknowledgments

Together we wish to thank all those colleagues who gave generously of their time to assist us in this undertaking. These include Drs. David Belmonte, Michael Fauman, Rachel Glick, John Greden, Michael Jibson, David Knesper, Daniel Maixner, Melvin McInnis, Kenneth Silk, and Jonathon Sugar from the University of Michigan Department of Psychiatry; Drs. Bruce Gimbel, David Beltzman, William Bucknam, Ellen Perrici, and Edwin Tobes from the St. Joseph Mercy Hospital Department of Psychiatry; Dr. Blake Casher of the Michigan State University Department of Psychiatry; and Dr. Michael Brooks from Brighton Hospital. Dr. Lewis Opler from NYU School of Medicine provided a number of helpful suggestions for the schizophrenia chapter. *Special* thanks is in order to Mickey Taylor, neuropsychiatrist *extraordinaire*, without whose encouragement and guidance this book would not have advanced from its infancy – a manual for local residents and students – to its present published form.

Our current colleagues at University of Michigan Hospital keep us sharp, always lend a helping hand, and make it a pleasure to come to work every day. These include Drs. David Belmonte, Oliver Cameron, Rachel Glick, Laura Hirshbein, Michael Jibson, David Knesper, Dan Maixner, Amy Rosinski, Lisa Seyfried, and Mickey Taylor. All of the staff – nurses, social workers, activity therapists, patient care workers, and administrative assistants – on Unit 9C, C/L, and in Psychiatric Emergency Services, keep us on task and still manage to do all of the hard work.

We both learn so much from the University of Michigan psychiatry residents and medical students, who keep us on our toes and allow us the enjoyment of teaching and the fulfillment of watching bright young people mature into caring clinicians.

Furthermore, we both feel it imperative to highlight the steady leadership of our department, for many years with Dr. John Greden and now with Dr. Gregory Dalack continuing at the helm. We acknowledge their role in this book's formation by noting that they have created and fostered an academic atmosphere in which we and our colleagues are constantly encouraged and inspired to do our best work.

Dr. Michael I. Casher

As an unabashed "old school" psychiatrist, my journey has been one in which I have been influenced not only by my associations with numerous teachers and colleagues over the years, but also by the many hours "spent" with inspiring members of our field who are known to me primarily through their writings. Some of those who have been important to me have passed on, leaving their imparted knowledge or their written works as legacies, while others are still guiding our field and gracing us with their astuteness and wisdom. Psychiatry is an endeavor that – by its very nature – honors tradition, even while it looks to its newest generation for the vitality that will keep our field relevant and vibrant. And it is in thinking about this "generativity" cycle that I view my wisest decision with regard to this book to be the co-authorship of my young colleague Joshua Bess. He brings Swarthmore-bred writing skills, recent-graduate energy and enthusiasm, and modern clinical sensibility.

My family – my wife Yang and children Lucy, Gabriel, and Jennifer – has provided indirect support for this book in the form of love and encouragement. They deserve special thanks as well for the patience and forbearance required when one's spouse or father is preoccupied with such a time-consuming project.

Dr. Joshua D. Bess

I must acknowledge that this manual started out as, and in many ways still is, Michael Casher's baby. I was honored to be asked to be his co-author. These exciting first years of my career have been substantially enriched by having him as a boss, mentor, colleague, and friend.

I have been blessed to have wise guides and close confidants along each part of my path from small-town kid to big-university psychiatrist. I would like to mention specifically Jody Pearl, Professor Felicia Dixon, Professor Ahamindra Jain, Professor Michael Riley, Professor Thomas Gest, Dr. Timothy Florence, Dr. Jennifer Seibert, Dr. Joshua Ehrlich, and Dr. Gregory Dalack. These individuals, and many others, have kept me from wandering too far astray.

Unwavering support and encouragement from my family, while growing up and through many years of education, gave me a solid foundation from which to grow into the person I am today. And while I have worked for the past year on this manual, my wife Krista, a primary care physician, has kept me centered and focused. With seemingly endless energy, she has also kept our three toddlers – Gavan, Lillian, and Jacob – warm, fed, and happy. They are my purpose and inspiration.

MIC and JDB

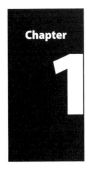

The inpatient with schizophrenia

When specific diagnoses are mentioned, we are referring to diagnoses and criteria as listed in the *Diagnostic and Statistical Manual of Mental Disorders*, 4th edition, text revision (DSM-IV-TR) unless otherwise specified.

Why might a patient with schizophrenia be admitted to a psychiatric unit?

Patients with schizophrenia who meet the criteria for admission to an inpatient unit are generally quite ill. The so-called "positive symptoms" of schizophrenia, which can result in threatening behavior and loss of control, are the usual triggers for admission. Some admitted patients will be experiencing a "first break," while others are hospitalized with an exacerbation of pre-existing schizophrenia. Most obvious symptoms are generally related to psychosis, a loss of reality testing and impaired mental functioning [1]. Psychosis usually presents with hallucinations, delusions, thought disorder, and/or bizarre or disruptive behavior (Table 1.1). The onset of illness or worsening of psychotic symptoms may be noticed by a family member, friend, teacher, co-worker, employer, or caregiver who sees the patient behaving bizarrely and deteriorating in their ability to function. A given patient may be so disruptive in the community that he or she is brought to the emergency department by police. A patient might even be hospitalized involuntarily for a time, depending on the laws and criteria in their state [2].

The negative symptoms of schizophrenia, such as social withdrawal and apathy, are very often also present in inpatients and contribute largely to the overall morbidity of the illness. However, these symptoms alone do not generally precipitate a stay on the inpatient unit unless they are so severe that patients are unable to adequately care for themselves outside of the hospital.

How does the inpatient clinician approach an interaction with an acutely psychotic patient?

Though it is important to establish a treatment alliance with a patient early in their stay, psychosis is often accompanied by lack of insight and

Table 1.1 Symptoms of psychosis

Symptom	Definition	Example
Hallucination	false sensory perception in the absence of actual input	auditory hallucination: for example hearing a man's voice commenting on one's actions
Delusion	false belief based on incorrect inference about external reality	paranoid delusion: for example belief that one's psychiatrist is attempting administer deadly poison
Thought disorder	disturbance of thinking that affects language and communication	loose associations: expressing unrelated ideas in succession without logical transitions or connections

neurocognitive deficits that hamper this process. Clinicians also need to be mindful of their own safety, which, with certain very agitated patients or patients with a known history of violence, might entail having one or more staff members or security officers either observe the interview or be on "standby" just outside. Also, a 2 mg dose of lorazepam is a wonderful adjunct to even the most soothing bedside manner! Early efforts are directed toward calming the patient sufficiently for the interview to proceed. When the patient is ready to participate, the interviewer's manner should be reassuring, calm, and non-judgmental. Patients can become more agitated if the interviewer appears incredulous or challenging when confronted with the patient's frankly delusional ideas (Table 1.2).

The following vignette illustrates the kind of flexibility that is necessary to engage these often distrustful individuals:

A young indigent woman, in her first episode of illness, presented to the psychiatric emergency department with a recent history of eating from dumpsters, as she feared she would be poisoned by the various church meals offered in the area. Once hospitalized, she would not take oral medication for the same reason, and thus required a court order for injectable medication. The treatment team eventually discovered that she was very worried about her inability to pay her student loans. When team members demonstrated their willingness to help her with this issue, assisting with loan deferral forms and a disability application, she was able to be more engaged in treatment and was then willing to try oral medication for psychotic symptoms.

Table 1.2 *In our experience...* Hints for approaching a fearful or agitated patient

Always pay attention to your safety. Look for signs that the patient is escalating: profanity, clenched fists, threatening posture or movements toward you.

Make sure the patient does not feel trapped or cornered in the interview space.

Include a staff member who knows or already has rapport with the patient.

Offer the patient something tangible (e.g., food or a blanket).

Start with, or use exclusively, simple, concrete questions.

Leading questions/statements are often helpful, e.g., "Many patients tell me they feel uncomfortable talking to a doctor about these experiences."

Keep your own affect display to a minimum.

Do not try to be overly friendly or familiar, even if you know the patient.

If necessary, keep the initial interview brief and return to complete your assessment later.

Don't focus solely on medications; they are often a source of contention, fear, or distrust.

Remember: No matter how nervous or frightened you are, the patient is much more so.

What historical information is important with a first-break patient?

Particular attention should be paid to time course and intensity of psychotic symptoms. However, early on, especially if time is limited, fully flushing out intricate details of complex delusional symptoms can be delayed to a later meeting. A detailed inquiry into use of illicit substances and alcohol is key, since not only is there a high co-morbidity of substance use with schizophrenia, but because substance intoxication and withdrawal are often causes of or contributors to psychosis [3]. The clinician should also carefully determine whether there are, or have been, any mood symptoms, since they are the deciding factor at a major fork in the diagnostic road.

A complete social history, which in most instances is best obtained from family, is a high priority. This will help to outline the longitudinal course of illness. One should find out when family members first noticed changes in their loved-ones' social, educational, or occupational functioning. Also, especially important here, is a complete developmental history. Schizophrenic patients are often "odd" kids or demonstrate prodromal symptoms during their teenage years. There is a much better prognosis in a patient who was fully functional six weeks before the admission compared to a patient who "never had any friends" and has experienced a slow deterioration over a period of years.

Table 1.3 *In our experience...* Hints for recognizing psychoses other than schizophrenia

Delusional disorder – can be high functioning with very circumscribed and believable false ideas. Staff on unit will sometimes debate if the patient is truly psychotic.

Shared delusional disorder – the "non-dominant" deluded partner may have some Axis II vulnerability or be in a very dependant relationship with the "true" psychotic partner

Brief psychotic disorder – look for a significant stressor in a vulnerable individual. Can be time-limited and remit without medications once in the structure of the hospital

Schizoaffective disorder – look for separation of the affective and psychotic components of illness. Tend to function better than pure schizophrenic patients.

Psychotic disorder due to medical illness – the physical examination, medical history, and laboratory tests can be crucial. More likely to have cognitive dysfunction or other signs of delirium.

Substance-induced psychotic disorder – look for other stigmata of drug or alcohol use and pay attention to the drug screen and markers for alcohol use.

Post-partum psychosis – look for confusion and disorganization in addition to delusions/hallucinations. Many have bipolar personal or family history. Also look for delusions/obsessions about the baby.

Remember: Not all people who are delusional have schizophrenia. Look for the nuances that rule the other possibilities in or out.

In the early stage of illness, such as with a "first break," it is important to try to pin down the most specific diagnosis possible. This has implications for prognosis, treatment, and the institution of social supports. That said, many experienced inpatient psychiatrists often discharge a patient with a considerable hedging on the final diagnosis, e.g., "Psychotic Disorder NOS, rule-out Schizophrenia." After all, an inpatient admission and the events leading up to it are only a small cross-section of a patient's life. Follow-up studies have demonstrated that experienced psychiatrists' provisional diagnosis of schizophrenia from an index admission "stays true" only one-half to two-thirds of the time. Psychiatrists should all become familiar with the other DSM illnesses classified under Schizophrenia and Other Psychotic Illnesses as they have differing courses, prognoses, and recommended treatments (Table 1.3).

What is the initial work-up of a psychotic patient?

A complete work-up for medical causes of psychosis ferrets out cases where a physical illness, possibly a curable one, presents with symptoms similar to schizophrenia. This work-up should include a urine drug screen, a

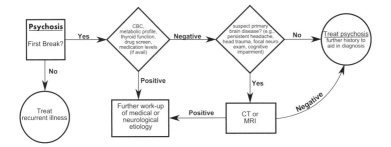

Figure 1.1 Initial work-up of first-break psychosis.

comprehensive metabolic laboratory profile, and thyroid functions. Some clinicians order a magnetic resonance imaging (MRI) or computed tomography (CT) scan of the brain in the instance of a first break, but more conservative guidelines reserve imaging for cases where there is some level of suspicion of a primary brain disease: presence of persistent headaches, history of head trauma, lateralizing findings on neurological examination, or significant cognitive impairment (Figure 1.1). Findings on the physical examination or mental status testing can also guide one toward a more extensive work-up, including lumbar puncture, electroencephalogram (EEG), heavy metals, copper and ceruloplasmin, etc. The involvement of a neurologist can be helpful if there are specific signs or symptoms that suggest the possibility of a primary neurological illness.

How does one distinguish psychosis in schizophrenia from mania in bipolar disorder?

This is a challenging differential diagnosis: a patient from either group can present in an enraged and/or paranoid state with persecutory and/or grandiose delusions. In the small snapshot one sees in the hospital, the states can be indistinguishable. But the pathway of each to psychotic symptoms differs. That is why longitudinal history from family and friends is extremely important in differentiating schizophrenia from bipolar disorder. In the months or years leading up to the psychotic break, schizophrenic patients will usually show a pattern of withdrawal and isolation, where bipolar patients can have periods of extra energy and hypomanic gregariousness. Depressive symptoms observed by loved-ones in this prodromal period, though important to note, do not always point to bipolar disorder, since the negative symptoms of schizophrenia often look like depression. If information about the patient's behaviors leading up to the current episode is unclear or unavailable, some clinicians find it useful to look at old family movies and photographs to see if the patient

Table 1.4 *In our experience*. . . Questions to help obtain family history in difficult cases

Was anyone in your family ever institutionalized? . . .in a state hospital? . . .in an asylum?
Were there relatives that went away for periods of time without explanation?
Did any of your relatives take pills for their nerves?
Did anyone in your family die unexpectedly? . . .without an explanation of how?
Did you ever hear of a family member getting shock treatments?
Was there a relative that your family avoided talking about?
Any relatives that other family members said were "funny," "not right," or "crazy?"

Remember: Diagnoses evolve. . . an uncle with "schizophrenia" in the 1950s might not meet the current criteria for that diagnosis.

appeared odd or ill at ease as a child, which turns out to be a harbinger of the development of schizophrenia in adolescence or early adulthood [4, 5].

Family history can also be helpful in making the distinction between these two categories of illness. A strong family history of any mood disorder, and especially a well described family history of bipolar disorder, can be combined with other observations to make a good case for the current patient having the same illness. Similarly, a pedigree that includes relatives with schizophrenia or schizophrenic spectrum disorders (e.g., schizotypal or schizoid features) can give *some* weight to the diagnosis of schizophrenia. However, a clinician must be careful when it comes to deciding how much emphasis to place on family history in the process of diagnosis, especially with schizophrenia. First, family history is often unreliable, with different relatives giving different information [6]. Also, while the concordance rate for identical twins is 80% in bipolar disorder, it is only 50% in schizophrenia [1]. In other words, the significance of a patient having a bipolar relative is greater than that of a schizophrenic relative (Table 1.4).

What factors are considered when a patient with known schizophrenia is admitted?

First, one needs to make sure the diagnosis is correct. While the field of psychiatry has made great strides in reliability and stability of diagnoses, especially schizophrenia, it is still far from 100% [7, 8]. The last provider observed the patient over just a brief length of time, just like the current provider is about to do when a patient is admitted.

When a patient with confirmed schizophrenia is admitted to the inpatient unit, the primary task of the inpatient team is to determine what circumstances led to decompensation [9]. The most frequent cause for relapse is suboptimal adherence to an outpatient medication regimen. In these cases it is useful to get an assessment of the patient's attitude toward his or her illness and toward medication, as denial of illness predisposes to poor medication adherence. In other cases there is a specific psychosocial trigger, such as the loss of a supportive figure or a change in work environment. Other possible social stressors include loss of domicile, intense family interactions, and financial uncertainty. It is helpful to look at the past record for similar instances of relapse to see if there is a repeating pattern of relapse during stressful life events. Finally, associated alcohol or substance use can undermine the effects of an adequate antipsychotic regimen. Sometimes, as in the vignette below, a psychotic family member has "induced" psychosis in a vulnerable patient:

A 20-year-old man with schizophrenia and several hospitalizations in the past was stable on medication until several weeks prior to his current stay in the hospital. He was admitted through the emergency department in an acutely agitated, paranoid state that left him unable to attend to his basic needs. In a family meeting on the unit, his mother presented as floridly delusional herself! She had no understanding of, or empathy for, her son's illness, and was convinced that his problems were due to an antibiotic he had taken as a child. The patient, in a pathologically symbiotic tie to his mother, had adopted her viewpoint, and in the process had lost all trust in the treatment team at his outpatient clinic. His mother's level of disorganization left his family life in chaos, and he was further distressed by his mother's constant refrain to him that he "was not psychotic." His situation left him little recourse other than a further retreat into psychosis.

What factors are involved in choosing an antipsychotic medication?

Most of the time, the first-line treatment will be an atypical antipsychotic (also known as a second-generation antipsychotic, SGA). First, attention must be paid to the history of medications that a patient has already tried, since there is no sense in "reinventing the wheel." Contacting the patient's current outpatient psychiatrist is extremely important, as this provider will likely have useful insight into the patient's history of medication responsiveness. Next, there are usually formulary constraints on medication choices as laid down by the insurance company, government, or other payer. Remaining factors in choosing an antipsychotic are patient preference, side-effect profile of the drug, and efficacy. Since the efficacy among the atypical antipsychotics is roughly

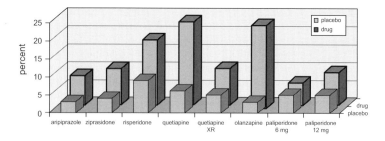

Figure 1.2 Percentage of patients with significant weight gain (>7%) in clinical studies [14–20].

equivalent [10], the choice among these medications really entails consideration of possible side effects. These include metabolic side effects – weight gain, hyperlipidemia, genesis of diabetes – that are at the fore of current research and monitoring efforts [11, 12, 13]; and also extra-pyramidal symptoms (EPS), orthostatic hypotension, activation/akathisia, and sedation (Figure 1.2 and Table 1.5). Determining which effects are most important to avoid for a given patient will go a long way toward improving adherence. With regard to patient preference, if a patient tells you "I'm not taking haldol!" (for example), he or she may be referring to past EPS or other reactions to haloperidol. Efforts should be made to find an alternative.

Further suggestions about medications:

1. If formulary restrictions or limited financial resources force the use of a first-generation, or typical, antipsychotic, consider a mid-potency drug such as perphenazine. This will steer a course between the relatively high EPS risk of the high-potency drugs (e.g., haloperidol) and the alpha blockade of the low-potency choices. The CATIE study, the CUtLASS study, and comparisons of the two, show near equivalence in efficacy for the traditional antipsychotics when compared with the atypical antipsychotics [28–31].

2. Still, atypical antipsychotics are the preferred medications under most circumstances. The overall side-effect burden is less than typical antipsychotics, with lower incidence of neuroleptic malignant syndrome, EPS and akathisia, and tardive dyskinesia [27]. Most psychiatrists place clozapine in a separate category, even among the atypicals. In some countries in South America and Europe, as well as in China, clozapine is in fact used as a first-line drug. In the United States clozapine is reserved for patients with refractory psychosis or severe tardive dyskinesia. Clozapine can be a god-send for these patients, and can significantly improve functioning. Unfortunately it requires extra monitoring, and has a significant risk of weight gain [32].

Table 1.5 Atypical antipsychotic *documented* side effects [13, 21–27, 33]

Medication[1]	Forms	Common side effects (≥5%, ≥15%)	Serious side effects (<1% but reported, ≥1%)
Clozapine	tablet, ODT	*Metabolic:* **weight gain (>50%),** diabetes	sudden cardiac death, QTc prolongation (no reports of TdP), myocarditis (rare), **syncope (5%), agranulocytosis (1.3%),** eosinophilia (1%), **neutropenia (3%), seizure (5%),** acute dystonia, NMS, tardive dyskinesia
		EPS: <5% overall	
		Other: **tachyarrhythmia (25%),** sweating, **excessive salivation (31%),** constipation, xerostomia, **dizziness (19%),** headache, **somnolence (39%),** tremor, **vertigo (19%)**	
Olanzapine	tablet, ODT, IR IM	*Metabolic:* **hypercholesterolemia (up to 24%), hyperglycemia (0.1% to 17.4%), increased appetite (24%), increased triglycerides (up to 40%), weight gain (up to 57%), diabetes**	QTc prolongation (no reports of TdP but report of VFib), **dystonic events (2% to 3%),** acute dystonia, NMS, tardive dyskinesia
		EPS: **overall 15–32%, parkinsonism 5% to 20%,** akathisia	
		Other: orthostatic hypotension, **increased prolactin (31.2% to 61.1%),** constipation, indigestion, xerostomia, **dizziness (4% to 18%),** insomnia, **somnolence (2% to 52%),** cough, rhinitis	

(continued)

Table 1.5 *(Continued)*

Medication[1]	Forms	Common side effects (≥5%, ≥15%)	Serious side effects (<1% but reported, ≥1%)
Risperidone[2]	tablet, ODT, solution, LA IM	*Metabolic:* **weight gain (up to 18%)**	sudden cardiac death, QTc prolongation w/ report(s) of TdP, **syncope (up to 2%)**, seizure, **dystonia (5–11%)**, NMS, tardive dyskinesia
		EPS: **overall 7% to 31%**, akathisia, **parkinsonism 0.6% to 20%**	
		Other: constipation, diarrhea, indigestion, nausea, **headache (15% to 21%)**, somnolence, tremor, **anxiety (2% to 16%)**, rhinitis	
Quetiapine	tablet, ER tablet	*Metabolic:* **increased cholesterol (9% to 16%), increased triglycerides (14% to 23%), weight gain (5% to 23%)**, increased appetite	QTc prolongation w/ report of TdP, **syncope (1%), leukopenia (at least 1% to 5%)**, neutropenia, seizure, acute dystonia, NMS, tardive dyskinesia
		EPS: overall 4% to 12%, tremor	
		Other: orthostatic hypotension, tachycardia, abdominal pain, constipation, indigestion, vomiting, **xerostomia (9% to 44%)**, increased liver enzymes, backache, asthenia, **dizziness (9% to 18%) headache (17% to 21%)**, insomnia, **sedation (30%), somnolence (16% to 34%), agitation (6% to 20%)**, pharyngitis, fatigue, pain	
Zotepine	tablet	*Metabolic:* **weight gain (28%)**	single report of QTc prolongation, **seizures (7% to 17%)**, acute dystonia, NMS, tardive dyskinesia

Medication[1] Forms		Common side effects (≥5%, ≥15%)	Serious side effects (<1% but reported, ≥1%)
		EPS: overall ~8%, **tremor (18%), akathisia (25%), rigidity (18%)**	
		Other: **insomnia (37%), constipation (10% to 39%), xerostomia (10% to 29%), somnolence (15% to 29%),** tachycardia, hypotension, rhinitis	
Amisulpride	tablet	*Metabolic:* **weight gain (18% to 21%)**	sudden death, QTc prolongation w/ report of TdP, acute dystonia, NMS, tardive dyskinesia
		EPS: **overall 12% to 26%,** hyperkinesia	
		Other: hypotension, somnolence, insomnia, anxiety, agitation, increased prolactin, galactorrhea	
Ziprasidone	capsule, IR IM	*Metabolic:* weight gain	QTc prolongation w/ report of TdP, acute dystonia, NMS, tardive dyskinesia
		EPS: **overall 14% to 31%,** akathisia, tremor, hypokinesis	
		Other: **orthostatic hypotension (frequent),** rash, constipation, diarrhea, indigestion, nausea, **dizziness (8% to 16%), somnolence (14% to 31%),** asthenia, **headache (18%)**	
Aripiprazole	tablet, solution, IR IM	*Metabolic:* **weight gain (2% to 30%)**	QTc prolongation (no reports of TdP), seizure, acute dystonia, NMS, tardive dyskinesia

(continued)

Table 1.5 *(Continued)*

Medication[1] Forms	Common side effects (≥5%, ≥15%)	Serious side effects (<1% but reported, ≥1%)
	EPS: **overall 2% to 27%, akathisia (2% to 25%),** tremor	
	Other: constipation, **nausea (8% to 15%),** vomiting, dizziness, **headache (12% to 27%), insomnia (8% to 18%),** sedation, **somnolence (5% to 26.3%),** blurred vision, **anxiety (4% to 17%),** restlessness, fatigue	
Paliperidone ER tablet	*Metabolic:* weight gain	QTc prolongation (no reports of TdP), acute dystonia, NMS, tardive dyskinesia
	EPS: overall 2% to 7%, akathisia, dystonia,	
	Other: tachyarrhythmia, **tachycardia (16%),[3] hyperprolactinemia (45% to 49%),[3]** dizziness,[3] headache, somnolence	
Iloperidone	*Metabolic:* **weight gain (1% to 18%)**	QTc prolongation (no reports of TdP), acute dystonia, NMS, tardive dyskinesia
	EPS: overall 4% to 5%	
	Other: orthostatic hypotension, tachycardia, **hyperprolactinemia (26%),** diarrhea, nausea, xerostomia, **dizziness (10% to 20%), somnolence (9% to 15%),** nasal congestion, fatigue	
Asenapine	*Metabolic:* weight gain	QTc prolongation (no reports of TdP), acute dystonia, NMS, tardive dyskinesia

Medication[1] Forms	Common side effects (≥5%, ≥**15%**)	Serious side effects (<1% but reported, ≥**1%**)
	EPS: overall 7–10%, akathisia	
	Other: **insomnia, somnolence**, nausea, anxiety, agitation	

[1]available in the US and/or UK; [2] does not include side-effect data in children; [3] observed in a geriatric sample; ODT = orally disintegrating tablet, ER = extended release, IR IM = immediate release intramuscular injection, LA IM = long-acting intramuscular injection, NMS = neuroleptic malignant syndrome, TdP = torsades de pointes

3. Long-acting depot injections are useful with patients who have difficulty with adherence to their medications, including those who are in court-mandated treatment. The side-effect profile of the depot formulations may actually be better than that of their oral counterparts, due to the lack of steep peaks in blood levels. An injection of haloperidol decanoate lasts three to four weeks and intramuscular (IM) fluphenazine decanoate lasts about two weeks. Long-acting IM risperidone is an alternative to those first-generation medications, *if* the patient has the means to pay for this expensive drug (~$10,000 per year) that is often not covered by health insurance. Some long-term patients require such high doses of typical antipsychotics in depot form that they can not be switched to long-acting risperidone and remain stable. However, for younger, more medication-naïve patients, the possible neurocognitive and side-effect advantages of risperidone over the traditional depot medications can be considerable.

What other medications are useful for inpatients with schizophrenia?

Although antipsychotics are the mainstay medications for schizophrenia, and are effective against the psychotic symptoms, there may be occasion for other classes of medications to be used during a patient's stay on the inpatient unit. Anti-anxiety medications (i.e., benzodiazepines) are often used acutely in conjunction with the antipsychotic to help calm very anxious or agitated patients.

Benzodiazepines are also are helpful for tremor or akathisia induced by the antipsychotics. Akathisia can be very distressing to patients and has been implicated as a possible contributor to suicide risk among people with schizophrenia [33]. Other medications used for akathisia include beta-blockers (e.g., propranolol) and anticholinergics (e.g., benztropine or trihexylphenidryl) (Table 1.6).

Table 1.6 Treatment options for akathisia [33]

Antipsychotic	lower dose
	switch to different agent
Adjunctive therapy (first line)	1. beta-blocker
	2. benzodiazepine
	3. anticholinergic
Adjunctive therapy (second line)	clonidine
	amantadine
	diphenhydramine
	serotonin antagonist
	mirtazapine
Psychosocial	patient education
	clear expectations
	open dialogue regarding risks
	reassurance

Other EPS, including dystonia, are usually initially treated with diphenhydramine, benztropine, or trihexylphenidryl. Amantadine is sometimes a useful adjunct.

Many patients with schizophrenia have co-morbid depressive symptoms, sometimes even severe enough to meet criteria for a co-occurring major depressive episode. If depressive symptoms are persistent, antidepressants can be useful. The first-line choice for depression in schizophrenia is usually a selective serotonin reuptake inhibitor (SSRI), mostly because of the side-effect profiles of older medications such as tricyclic antidepressants and monoamine oxidase inhibitors (MAOIs). But attention needs to be paid to possible interactions between the antidepressant and the antipsychotic, especially with respect to metabolism via the Cytochrome P450 (CYP-450) system. Fluoxetine and paroxetine are notorious inhibitors of several P-450 pathways, and can therefore increase the serum concentration of an antipsychotic, even to the point of toxicity. In terms of other antidepressants, trazodone or mirtazapine may be used off label as sleep aids while patients stabilize.

Patients with a significant aggressive or impulsive component to their schizophrenia, or with mood lability bordering on bipolar disorder, may benefit from addition of a mood stabilizer such as valproate, lithium, or carbamazepine. Again, monitoring of drug–drug interactions is important with this departure from monotherapy.

How do you manage the acutely agitated schizophrenic inpatient?

Threatening or violent behavior demands aggressive treatment on the inpatient unit to avoid injuries to staff or patient. The paranoia and hallucinations associated with schizophrenia can lead to a high degree of agitation. Staff must be trained in behavioral/verbal techniques for de-escalating patients. Seclusion and/or restraints are final resorts – reserved for imminent threat of the patient acting out in a dangerous manner, or after the patient has already lost control.

Aggressive use of pharmacotherapy can soothe a highly agitated patient and can prevent injury to patients and staff [34, 35]. Many psychiatrists still order the combination of haloperidol (5–10 mg) and lorazepam (1–2 mg). This is given IM every two to four hours until the patient is calm. There is a risk of EPS or dystonia, especially in younger patients, which would require the addition of benztropine or diphenhydramine to the regimen. More recently, second-generation antipsychotic medications have been used more frequently for management of acute agitation. Compared to traditional antipsychotics, these medicines have a lower incidence of adverse effects, including EPS/akathisia, dystonia, and neuroleptic malignant syndrome. Most commonly used are ziprasidone IM and olanzapine in IM or orally disintegrating form. Many hospital units are now using agitation protocols with associated rating scales such as the Behavioral Activity Rating Scale or the Positive and Negative Syndrome Scale (PANSS) agitation subscale to determine when patients require these aggressive medication regimens (Figure 1.3) [36, 37].

How do you evaluate and manage suicide risk in patients with schizophrenia on the inpatient unit?

Schizophrenia can lead to suicidal behavior through several mechanisms: response to command hallucinations, demoralization with the course of illness, associated depression, or disorganization of thought and action seen in psychosis. Patients should be monitored closely and evaluated for suicidal ideation, intent, and planning on a daily basis during the early part of the stay in the hospital. Furthermore, careful assessment of suicide risk is necessary every time privileges are advanced and at the time of discharge. Evaluation of suicidal thoughts and behavior on an inpatient unit includes consideration of demographic risk factors and protective factors (e.g., race, age, family history), acute or dynamic factors that can be addressed and mitigated during a patient's stay (e.g., social upheaval or command hallucinations), and detailed inquiry into suicidal ideation, plans, and behaviors while on the unit. A formal assessment tool can be useful, but does not replace a sound clinical evaluation. Young men with schizophrenia and a pre-morbid history of successful functioning are at particular risk for demoralization and suicide as they become

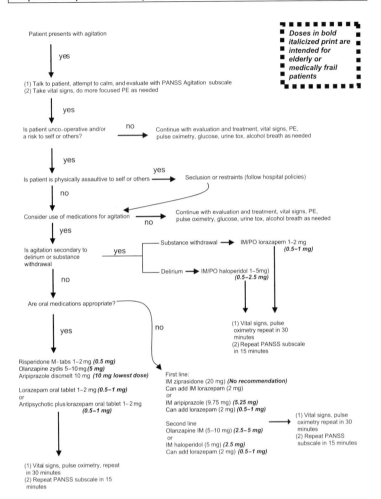

Figure 1.3 University of Michigan Inpatient Psychiatry Agitation Protocol.

cognizant of their decreased abilities and diminished prospects for fulfilling their aspirations [38, 39].

Antidepressants have a role in all of these instances if they do not resolve with treatment of psychosis. In addition, clozapine treatment has also been associated with a decrease in suicidal behaviors. It is the only antipsychotic with an indication from the United States Food and Drug Administration (FDA) for reducing the risk of recurrent suicidal behavior in patients with schizophrenia.

What is the overall treatment plan for patients with schizophrenia in the hospital?

Patients with schizophrenia first need relief from the acute psychosis and stabilization of the social circumstances that led to their hospitalization. The former is generally accomplished using the medications listed above. In the early phases of an inpatient stay, one should have brief interactions with the patient to assess their response to medication, especially focusing on side effects and other limitations to adherence. The general attitude toward the patient should be friendly and reassuring. Simple explanations work best since many schizophrenic patients have cognitive limitations and do not tolerate complicated didactic interactions. Once the patient begins to improve, he or she should be encouraged to attend group sessions and other activities on the unit. This is where the staff can assess overall level of functioning and help the patient reintegrate back to "normal life." Ideally there should be programming, groups, and/or activities on the unit that are specifically aimed at the functional level and treatment needs of patients with schizophrenia.

As psychotic symptoms improve, some patients will be able to benefit from discussions about the circumstances leading to hospitalization and what steps can be taken to prevent recurrences of illness. This should involve counseling about the need to abstain from drugs and alcohol, including referral to dual-diagnosis treatment if indicated, the need for regular sleep, and the need to adhere to medication regimen and follow-up appointments. Problem solving around job and family issues is also important. Interventions here might center on creating an environment for the patient that is free of unwarranted criticisms and unrealistic expectations that can easily destabilize the patient and lead to readmission.

A smooth transition from the hospital to outpatient treatment is essential, and is often difficult for patients who do not fully understand or accept their illness or the need for medication. Frequently patients with schizophrenia have such poor insight that court-ordered outpatient treatment is necessary. The latter part of the hospital stay can focus on setting up the outpatient appointments and adjusting the outpatient treatment plan, for example by adding psychotherapy, arranging a different housing situation, scheduling more frequent visits by an outreach team, or replacing oral medication with an injectable depot formulation.

References

1. Sadock B J, Sadock V A & Kaplan H I. *Kaplan & Sadock's Comprehensive Textbook of Psychiatry*, 8th edn. Philadelphia, PA: Lippincott Williams & Wilkins; 2004.

2. Treatment Advocacy Center. State standards for assisted treatment: state by state chart. September 2008; www.treatmentadvocacycenter.org [Accessed September 23, 2009].

3. Caton C L, Drake R E, Hasin D S *et al.* Differences between early-phase primary psychotic disorders with concurrent substance use and substance-induced psychoses. *Archives of General Psychiatry*, **62** (2) (2005), 137–45.

4. Walker E F, Grimes K E, Davis D M & Smith A J. Childhood precursors of schizophrenia: facial expressions of emotion. *American Journal of Psychiatry*, **150**:11 (1993), 1654–60.

5. Walker E F, Lewine R R & Neumann C. Childhood behavioral characteristics and adult brain morphology in schizophrenia. *Schizophrenia Research*, **22**:2 (1996), 93–101.

6. Roy M A, Walsh D & Kendler K S. Accuracies and inaccuracies of the family history method: a multivariate approach. *Acta Psychiatrica Scandinavica*, **93**:4 (1996) 224–34.

7. Haahr U, Friis S, Larsen T K *et al.* First-episode psychosis: diagnostic stability over one and two years. *Psychopathology*, **41**:5 (2008), 322–9.

8. Cheniaux E, Landeira-Fernandez J & Versiani M. The diagnoses of schizophrenia, schizoaffective disorder, bipolar disorder and unipolar depression: interrater reliability and congruence between DSM-IV and ICD-10. *Psychopathology*, **42**:5 (2009), 293–8.

9. Ayuso-Gutiérrez J L & del Río Vega J M. Factors influencing relapse in the long-term course of schizophrenia. *Schizophrenia Research*, **28**:2–3 (1997), 199–206.

10. Leucht S, Komossa K, Rummel-Kluge C *et al.* A meta-analysis of head-to-head comparisons of second-generation antipsychotics in the treatment of schizophrenia. *American Journal of Psychiatry*, **166**:2 (2009), 152–63.

11. American Diabetes Association, American Psychiatric Association, American Association of Clinical Endocrinologists, North American Association for the Study of Obesity. Consensus development conference on antipsychotic drugs and obesity and diabetes. *Diabetes Care*, **27**:2 (2004), 596–601.

12. Henderson D C. Weight gain with atypical antipsychotics: evidence and insights. *Journal of Clinical Psychiatry*, **68**:Suppl. 12 (2007), 18–26.

13. Newcomer J W. Second-generation (atypical) antipsychotics and metabolic effects: a comprehensive literature review. *CNS Drugs*, **19**:Suppl. 1 (2005), 1–93.

14. Invega [package insert]. Titusville, NJ: Ortho-McNeil-Janssen Pharmaceuticals, Inc., 2009.

15. Risperdal [package insert]. Titusville, NJ: Ortho-McNeil-Janssen Pharmaceuticals, Inc., 2009.

16. Abilify [package insert]. Tokyo: Otsuka Pharmaceutical Co, Ltd., 2009.

17. Seroquel XR [package insert]. Wilmington, DE: AstraZeneca Pharmaceuticals LP, 2009.

18. Seroquel [package insert]. Wilmington, DE: AstraZeneca Pharmaceuticals LP, 2009.

19. Geodon [package insert]. New York, NY: Pfizer, Inc., 2009.

20. Zyprexa [package insert]. Indianapolis, IN: Eli Lilly and Company, 2009.

21. Briffa D & Meehan T. Weight changes during clozapine treatment. *Australia and New Zealand Journal of Psychiatry*, **32**:5 (1998), 718–21.

22. Prakash A & Lamb H M. Zotepine: a review of its pharmacodynamic and pharmacokinetic properties and therapeutic efficacy in the management of schizophrenia. *CNS Drugs*, **9**:2 (1998), 153–75.

23. Brown C S, Farmer R G, Soberman J E & Eichner S F. Pharmacokinetic factors in the adverse cardiovascular effects of antipsychotic drugs. *Clinical Pharmacokinetics*, **43**:1 (2004), 33–56.

24. McKeage K & Plosker G L. Amisulpride: a review of its use in the management of schizophrenia. *CNS Drugs*, **18**:13 (2004), 933–56.

25. Stollberger C, Huber J O & Finsterer J. Antipsychotic drugs and QT prolongation. *International Clinical Psychopharmacology*, **20**:5 (2005), 243–51.

26. Bishara D & Taylor D. Upcoming agents for the treatment of schizophrenia: mechanism of action, efficacy and tolerability. *Drugs*, **68**:16 (2008), 2269–92.

27. DRUGDEX® System. www.thomsonhc.com [Accessed October 3, 2009].

28. Haddad P M & Dursun S. Selecting antipsychotics in schizophrenia: lessons from CATIE. *Journal of Psychopharmacology*, **20**:3 (2006), 332–4.

29. Jones P B, Barnes T R E, Davies L *et al*. Randomized controlled trial of the effect on quality of life of second- vs first-generation antipsychotic drugs in schizophrenia: cost utility of the latest antipsychotic drugs in schizophrenia study (CUtLASS 1). *Archives of General Psychiatry*, **63**:10 (2006), 1079–87.

30. Lewis S & Lieberman J. CATIE and CUtLASS: can we handle the truth? *British Journal of Psychiatry*. **192**:3 (2008), 161–3.

31. Lieberman J A, Stroup T S, McEvoy J P *et al*. Effectiveness of antipsychotic drugs in patients with chronic schizophrenia. *New England Journal of Medicine*, **353**:12 (2005), 1209–23.

32. Lieberman J A & Tasman A. *Handbook of Psychiatric Drugs*. Chichester, England; Hoboken, NJ: John Wiley & Sons; 2006.

33. Kane J M, Fleischhacker W W, Hansen L *et al*. Akathisia: an updated review focusing on second-generation antipsychotics. *Journal of Clinical Psychiatry*, **70**:5 (2009), 627–43.

34. Citrome L. Agitation III: Pharmacologic treatment of agitation. In: Glick R L, Berlin J S, Fishkind A B & Zeller S L, eds. *Emergency Psychiatry: Principles and Practice*. Philadelphia, PA: Wolters Kluwer Health/Lippincott Williams & Wilkins; 2008.

35. Battaglia J. Pharmacological management of acute agitation. *Drugs*, **65**:9 (2005), 1207–22.

36. Kay S R, Fiszbein A & Opler L A. The positive and negative syndrome scale (PANSS) for schizophrenia. *Schizophrenia Bulletin*, **13**:2 (1987), 261–76.

37. Swift R H, Harrigan E P, Cappelleri J C, Kramer D & Chandler L P. Validation of the behavioural activity rating scale (BARS): a novel measure of activity in agitated patients. *Journal of Psychiatric Research*, **36**:2 (2002), 87–95.

38. Bourgeois M, Swendsen J, Young F *et al*. Awareness of disorder and suicide risk in the treatment of schizophrenia: results of the international suicide prevention trial. *American Journal of Psychiatry*, **161**:8 (2004), 1494–6.

39. Clarke M, Whitty P, Browne S *et al*. Suicidality in first episode psychosis. *Schizophrenia Research*, **86**:1–3 (2006), 221–5.

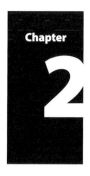

The inpatient with depression

When specific diagnoses are mentioned, we are referring to diagnoses and criteria as listed in the *Diagnostic and Statistical Manual of Mental Disorders*, 4th edition, text revision (DSM-IV-TR) unless otherwise specified.

What circumstances lead to hospitalization of a patient with depression?

Most patients with uncomplicated depression can be treated as an outpatient. Inpatient care is generally reserved for people with severe or treatment-resistant depressive symptoms, high suicide risk, and/or impaired self-care [1]. These are patients whose initial presentation is so severe as to warrant hospitalization, or who have "failed" outpatient treatment. In both cases the inpatient provider must complete a full diagnostic and therapeutic assessment. Even with patients who already have an outpatient team, the inpatient psychiatrist should be prepared to reevaluate the diagnosis and overall plan since the patient is not responding well to outpatient treatment.

Patients are frequently admitted to initiate a course of electroconvulsive therapy (ECT) [2]. Even though some patients who require ECT have the necessary support from their outpatient treatment team and their loved ones to negate the need for admission based on their illness alone, this treatment requires some diagnostic testing and co-ordination of care that is usually most efficiently done in the hospital. Furthermore, patients' initial tolerance of the procedure and possible early response can be observed and adjustments can be made to the treatment course as necessary.

Another factor involved in the decision to admit to a psychiatric unit is one or more significant co-morbid medical conditions. It may be safer to treat a medically-fragile person with severe depression on an inpatient unit, where responses to medications can be closely monitored. An example of this would be a person with coronary disease who requires psychotropic medications with potential cardiovascular side effects.

Finally, level of social support can be a major factor in the choice between ongoing outpatient care and admission to the hospital. A solid support network can allow even very ill patients to remain safe in outpatient treatment. For example, a devoted spouse may be able to keep medications and weapons out of the hands of a suicidal patient. In the absence of this level of support, though, a patient who is intensely suicidal will need the physical protection and staff interventions available on an inpatient unit.

What are general issues in initial evaluation and treatment of depression on the inpatient unit?

The hospitalization of a depressed patient is often the culmination of a severe crisis in the patient's life, leading to a temporary inability to function without structure and support. Patients will often view this as humiliating and shameful, or representing personal failure on their part [3]. This cognitive distortion should be discouraged, with emphasis placed on the opportunity for careful assessment and aggressive treatment, in addition to increased insight and emotional growth.

The biopsychosocial model – a philosophy of clinical care that takes into account the biological, psychological, *and* social aspects of a patient's illness – is a powerful way to conceptualize a case and can be useful in formulating a comprehensive treatment plan [4, 5]. This approach reminds clinicians to consider the relative contributions of not only genetic predisposition and biological substrates of illness, but also temperament, psychological factors, social stressors, and environment. When one of the three is particularly prominent, it is tempting to neglect the balance. Even in the case of a severely depressed, melancholic patient with multiple episodes of illness and strong genetic loading for affective disorders, a clinician must realize that grief and loss issues and lack of social support can still play a major role in sustaining depressed mood.

Some patients, even with severe depression, improve markedly within a few days on the inpatient unit. How can this be? The response time for most antidepressants is several weeks! Patients also respond to non-pharmacologic elements inherent in an inpatient stay: instilling of hope through the process of admission, respite from stress at home and work, validation and endorsement for a temporary "sick role," the kindness and support of the staff, and the concentrated therapeutic groups and activities [6]. Improvement in sleep through brief use of sleep aids, and attention to nutritional status also play a role. Hospitalization in and of itself is a major intervention with powerful effects. However, care needs to be taken so that this early improvement is not used to justify a premature discharge before an in-depth assessment of the patient is completed. Sometimes this early improvement is precarious and a more prolonged stay with aggressive medication adjustments or ECT will be needed.

What about involuntary hospitalizations?

When a depressed patient lacks insight into the need for treatment, an involuntary hospitalization may be necessary [7]. One common scenario is the depressed patient who has a serious overdose and is admitted to a general medical floor. The psychiatric consultation/liaison team will be called upon to evaluate the patient for psychiatric hospitalization. From a diagnostic perspective, the patient may be suffering from any of a number of forms of depression, ranging from serious Major Depressive Disorder with Melancholic Features to Adjustment Disorder with Depressed Mood. If the psychiatric team assesses that the patient requires a psychiatric stay, and the patient refuses to be voluntarily admitted, the team must then assess whether the patient meets the criteria for civil commitment [8]. In most states in the United States, these criteria include a substantial disorder of thought or mood, accompanied by "clear and convincing evidence" of dangerousness to self or others, or inability to care for self. Laws governing commitment, a.k.a. "sectioning," in the UK are similar.

One of two arguments is usually made in order to support civil commitment of the depressed patient, as in the example above. First, sometimes it is evident from examination of the patient that he/she does not have any insight into the potential lethality of the act just committed. While this lack of insight may weaken the assertion that the overdose was "really a suicide attempt" in the first place, it also points to a lower threshold for a repeat action in the near future. The second argument rests on the assumption that if the depressive symptoms are severe, the patient is unable to make the reasonable decisions that she/he would normally make when not so impaired by the symptoms.

What should be covered during the admission interview?

Psychiatric inpatients admitted for "depression" may be in the depressive phase of Bipolar Disorder or having a depressive reaction to a situation, such as in Adjustment Disorder with Depressed Mood. Inpatient units also see patients who meet criteria for Mood Disorder Due to a General Medical Condition or Substance-Induced Mood Disorder. Most of the rest of the depressed patients admitted to an inpatient unit will meet DSM-IV-TR criteria for a Major Depressive Episode (Table 2.1, Figure 2.1). A patient must have five of the nine symptoms listed for two weeks, including at least one of the first two symptoms (depressed mood or loss of interest or pleasure). Symptoms must cause distress and impairment in functioning. Also the symptoms cannot be part of a mixed state or due to substances, a general medical condition, or bereavement. An important duty of the inpatient team is to classify the depression as specifically as possible, since it will have implications for the treatment plan. It is especially important to recognize subtypes of depression such as melancholic features, catatonic features, and/or psychotic features, since there are special treatment considerations with each of these groupings (see below).

The mnemonic "SIG: E-CAPS" (Table 2.2) [9], developed by Carey Gross MD for Massachusetts General Hospital psychiatry residents, is very useful in

Table 2.1 DSM-IV-TR criteria for Major Depression (abbreviated)

Depressed mood most of the day, nearly every day

Markedly diminished interest or pleasure in activities

Significant weight loss or weight gain

Insomnia or hypersomnia

Psychomotor agitation or retardation

Fatigue or loss of energy

Feelings of worthlessness or guilt

Decreased concentration or indecisiveness

Recurrent thoughts of death; suicidal ideation, plans or attempts

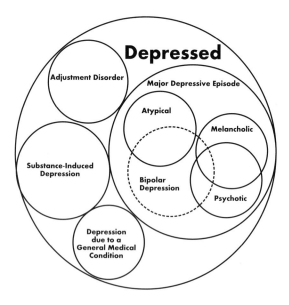

Figure 2.1 Various diagnoses that can present with "depression."

recalling the eight neurovegetative symptoms of depression. But, it is not refined enough for a detailed probing of a patient's depressive experience and consequent treatment planning. A more detailed rating scale, such as the Hamilton Rating Scale for Depression (HAM-D), the Beck Depression

Table 2.2 SIG: E-CAPS, a mnemonic for symptoms of depression

S	Suicidal thoughts
I	Interests decreased (anhedonia)
G	Guilt
E	Energy decreased
C	Concentration decreased
A	Appetite disturbance (increased or decreased)
P	Psychomotor changes (agitation or retardation)
S	Sleep disturbance (increased or decreased)

Inventory (BDI), or the Montgomery-Asberg Depression Rating Scale (MADRS) can be incorporated into the work-up and ongoing monitoring of inpatients with depression [10]. Rating scales are also useful tools for helping residents and students gain greater precision in the evaluation of depressive symptoms.

Going "beyond the DSM," [11] the inpatient clinician should inquire about a patient's level of social withdrawal or isolation. How many hours per day is the patient lying on the couch or retreating to bed? How many hours are spent in a productive fashion? If a patient reports crying episodes, the clinician must explore how often these occur and how long they last. A good history includes questions about how symptoms fluctuate through the day. Diurnal variation, with more severe symptoms in the morning, is a hallmark of "biological" depression. Attention must also be paid to the possibility of accompanying psychotic symptoms, most commonly nihilistic delusions, delusions of poverty, and somatic delusions.

How does one assess for melancholic depression?

The melancholic subtype of depression is overrepresented on the inpatient unit, especially among the treatment-resistant group (Table 2.3) [12]. These patients have more "biological" features of depression, including vegetative/motor disturbances, cognitive impairment (pseudodementia), and abnormal biological markers involving the hypothalamic–pituitary axis (HPA) [13, 14]. Melancholic depression may be poorly responsive to selective serotonin reuptake inhibitors (SSRIs), serotonin and norepinephrine reuptake inhibitors (SNRIs), and psychotherapy, but respond favorably to tricyclic antidepressants (TCAs) and/or ECT [15, 16]. Taylor and Fink (2008) have argued that melancholia should be considered a separate diagnosis. They propose a set of criteria different from, but overlapping with DSM-IV-TR (Table 2.4) [17]. It

Table 2.3 DSM-IV-TR criteria for Melancholic Features Specifier [18]

Either of the following, occurring during the most severe period of the current episode:

Loss of pleasure in all, or almost all, activities

Lack of reactivity to usually pleasurable stimuli (does not feel much better, even temporarily, when something good happens)

AND three (or more) of the following:

Distinct quality of depressed mood (i.e., the depressed mood is experienced as distinctly different from the kind of feeling experienced after the death of a loved one)

Depression regularly worse in the morning

Early morning awakening (at least two hours before usual time of awakening)

Marked psychomotor retardation or agitation

Significant anorexia or weight loss

Excessive or inappropriate guilt

Table 2.4 Criteria for Melancholia proposed by Fink and Taylor [19]

Disturbed mood of apprehension, worry or despondency

Psychomotor disturbance of agitation, retardation (including stupor and catatonia) or both

At least two vegetative signs: poor sleep, appetite, libido, cognition

At least one of the following:

Abnormal dexamethasone suppression test/high night-time cortisol level

Decreased REM latency or other sleep abnormalities

is important to recognize this pathology quickly in order to intervene as soon as possible (Table 2.5, Figure 2.2).

What are some of the special considerations in evaluating women with depression?

Recent research suggests that pre-menopausal women are more likely to have atypical features when suffering from depression. These woman also respond better to SSRIs or monoamine oxidase inhibitors (MAOIs) than TCAs [14]. In some women, there are hormonal correlates of depressive mood, which lead to

Table 2.5 *In our experience...* Clues for melancholic depression on the inpatient unit

The "omega sign" (see furrowed-browed figure in Figure 2.2)

Difficulty remembering happy times

Loved ones very aware of patient's level of suffering

Pacing the hallways, especially in the morning

Excessive worry about paying the hospital bill, being a burden on family or staff

Rare attendance at groups, activities

Poor participation in milieu

Remember: Distinguishing between "sick" and "not sick" is important in psychiatry, too!

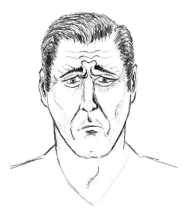

Figure 2.2 Illustration of the "omega sign" and other visible clues to melancholic depression. Drawn by Vasilis Pozios MD.

variations in mood with the menstrual cycle or to post-partum depression. Women with a history of severe premenstrual syndrome, premenstrual dysphoric disorder, or post-partum depression are at risk for developing peri-menopausal depression [20]. Moreover, post-menopausal depression in women is more likely to be of the melancholic sub-type, with particularly strong HPA alteration [14].

Of course, an inpatient clinician needs to be alert to the possibility that a female patient is currently pregnant. This would have implications for medication choices and therapeutic approach. A screening urine pregnancy test is an important part of the initial inpatient evaluation of a woman of child-bearing age.

What style should the interviewer adopt in the initial interview?

An important function of the initial interview is to develop rapport with the patient and to learn about him or her "as a person" outside of the diagnosis. Patients need a chance to "tell their story" and accordingly, the clinician should allow interview time for a departure from the recitation of symptoms, and explore, for instance, the patient's upbringing, current worries, or important relationships [21]. A more relaxed interview is more likely to foster a trusting therapeutic relationship, which is key to encouraging adherence to any treatment plan [22]. Moreover, a solid rapport allows the patient to discuss emotionally difficult issues – such as childhood abuse, current abuse, or occult substance use – that might have a large impact on the diagnostic assessment and treatment planning.

What is the role of family in providing history?

Family members should be enlisted to corroborate or fill in details of a patient's depressive history. Involvement of family is especially important when the patient is elderly. These patients sometimes do not feel "sad," [23, 24] are cognitively impaired [25], are too physically debilitated to give an adequate history, or are consciously denying symptoms in order to avoid admission or further hospitalization. Family may also help define the time-line of the patient's depression, i.e., was it an insidious process or did it come on suddenly? Family members are also better positioned to recall an early onset of depression in childhood. This is very important, since the onset of depression prior to age 11 is associated with a high probability of a subsequent development of adult bipolar disorder [26]. Finally, family members usually have special insights into the patient's long-term functioning history, temperament, and psychological make-up. These insights are invaluable in the overall evaluation and treatment planning for the patient.

All of the above notwithstanding, cautious comparison of information from all sources is important. There is often disagreement between collateral informants and the patient [25].

What about "other" causes of depression?

This is an *especially* important issue on the inpatient psychiatry unit. A thorough general medical evaluation must be part of every inpatient psychiatric assessment. There are a number of general medical and neurological conditions that can present as depression [27] (see Table 2.8). (One common adult psychiatry board question involves the occurrence of depression associated with pancreatic cancer, in which the mood disorder can actually precede any physical manifestation of illness.) Routine laboratory testing (comprehensive metabolic profile, complete blood count with differential, urine analysis, and thyroid function) should be included in the overall evaluation, with more detailed testing performed if the examination or history suggests a medically related cause for depression. A blood alcohol level and urine drug screen can help to assess for occult substance use as a cause for depression and/or poor response to treatment.

Imaging studies, usually computed tomography (CT) or magnetic resonance imaging (MRI), can be useful in some circumstances. However, research to clearly support widespread screening with neuro-imaging in depression is lacking since findings have been mixed and of questionable clinical utility [28–31]. Imaging should be reserved for particular situations where one has reasonable suspicion for a secondary cause or serious co-morbidity, such as severely treatment-resistant melancholic depression, possible dementia-related depression, or peculiar symptoms that do not match a typical depressive picture. Neuro-imaging can also be considered for depressed patients with severe avolitional states, frank catatonia, and/or frontal signs. Patients with specific or lateralizing findings on neurological examination or new, sudden onset of symptoms should also be considered for imaging, as shown in the following dramatic cases:

A 25-year-old woman presented with severe melancholic depression. In addition, she reported recent onset of severe headaches. An MRI scan revealed a frontal mass that turned out to be a cryptococcal abscess. After evacuation of the infection and a course of intravenous antibiotics, the patient's mood disorder completely resolved.

A 38-year-old woman was admitted to the inpatient unit with catatonic signs, fecal incontinence, and a high degree of amotivation. She had become depressed soon after the birth of her first child two years previously, and was pregnant with her second child at the time of admission. Initially the team thought she had some version of post-partum depression. But the astute resident, puzzled by the unusual presentation, ordered a CT scan. The scan showed a left frontal meningioma. Surgical removal of the tumor led to remission of her depression.

Neuropsychological testing should be considered when significant deficits in cognitive testing or cognitive processing are detected in a depressed inpatient. Signs of non-dominant hemispheric dysfunction include visual–spatial problems and apraxia; while dominant hemispheric problems would include word-finding difficulty. Though some degree of cognitive impairment can be part of severe depression (so-called pseudodementia), this finding can also represent a primary brain disorder, including dementias, seizure disorders, or sequelae of past head injury. Besides imaging tests discussed above, electro-encephalogram (EEG) and/or neurology consultation can be helpful in detecting these causes of depression.

How should the inpatient clinician evaluate patients' suicidal thoughts?

A 50-year-old man, admitted to the medical unit for treatment of cellulitis, was assessed by the psychiatry consultation-liaison service. The patient's first remark to the psychiatry resident was "Did you hear about that elevator accident? I caused it." In truth, there had been no such accident! The resident found that the patient had a number of symptoms consistent with depression in, addition to this delusional guilt. The gentleman was ultimately admitted to the psychiatric unit. There he committed suicide. Reviewing the case afterward, it seemed that since this delusional patient felt responsible for the deaths of others he then felt the need to punish himself.

This above case illustrates the need to do a detailed suicide assessment on all patients with depression. Sure, patients are admitted to the hospital to be kept safe, but several dozen commit suicide on inpatient psychiatric units in the United States every year [32]. There should be frequent follow-up assessments, especially during transition points in the hospitalization – e.g., increase in privileges, a stressful therapy session, a family meeting, or at discharge [32, 33]. Discharge is not only a stressful time for the patient, but is of course the time when the team must carefully weigh the risk of imminent suicide against the benefit of transitioning the patient to a lower level of care. Of note, several studies have shown that up to 65% of patients who commit suicide have been admitted to a psychiatric unit within the past year; around 10% of those who complete a suicide attempt do so on the day of discharge [34–36]. In summary, virtually all patients with depression on an inpatient unit are at *some* risk for suicide, with the periods of highest risk just after admission, during changes in privileges, and soon after discharge.

A comprehensive suicide assessment should include notice of demographic risk factors [37, 38], keeping in mind that people who commit suicide in the hospital "look" different than the high-risk individuals in the general population [39, 40]. Close attention must be paid to key symptoms of perturbation (e.g., psychosis, especially delusions and command hallucinations, in addition to anxiety and agitation) [33]. These symptoms are associated with significant suicide risk, and are often under-treated, even in the hospital (Table 2.6).

Table 2.6 Suicide risk factors in depressed patients on the inpatient unit

Acute (very responsive to inpatient mental health interventions)	psychosis (especially command hallucinations)
	anxiety and/or panic
	insomnia
	agitation
	delirium
	pain/discomfort from acute illness
	substance intoxication or withdrawal
	availability of means (with special attention to guns)
Sub-acute (responsive to mental health interventions, but brief inpatient admission not likely enough)	hopelessness/helplessness
	detailed suicide plan
	alcohol or substance use disorder
	withdrawing from loved ones
	anger
	bereavement +/– "reunion fantasy"
Environmental (changes take significant time, likely require efforts by others in addition to patient)	chronic medical illness, chronic pain
	lack of social support
	abusive relationship
	triggering events that evoke shame or despair
	poor finances
	legal trouble
	impending or recent end of relationship (death, divorce, etc.)
Demographic or static (cannot be changed)	suicide attempt that led to admission
	history of past suicide attempts
	history of trauma
	family history of suicide
	anniversary of traumas or losses
	age, race, gender

A history of alcohol or substance use, previous suicide attempts, family history of suicides, anniversaries of traumas, and current environmental factors triggering despair and/or shame are also important areas to assess. Examples of factors in the last category would be financial difficulty, chronic pain, or lack of interpersonal support. A detailed inquiry into the patient's thoughts, plans, behaviors, and intent with regard to self-harm must also be included, but *by no means* is the only piece of the puzzle. The prospective study by Busch and colleagues found that "77% of the patients…who took their lives while in the hospital denied suicidal ideation at their last recorded communication" [33]. On the other hand, Powell *et al.* found that suicidal plan or act of self-harm leading to/during admission – in addition to delusions, chronic mental illness, a first-degree relative who committed suicide, and recent bereavement – were strongly predictive of inpatient suicide in a study of 97 events over 30 years in four English counties [39]. Finally, access to means, especially availability of firearms, which should be removed from the home prior to a patient's discharge, should be reviewed [41].

A provider also needs to examine closely for factors that *may* decrease the patient's risk for suicide. These could include religious beliefs that proscribe suicidal acts; responsibilities and commitments to family and friends (especially children); a good treatment alliance with outpatient providers; and/or a safety plan [42, 43]. However, although recent literature refers to these items as "protective factors," they merely decrease risk somewhat – the risk is still present. In the words of a close colleague of the authors, "A depressed, psychotic, Catholic woman with two small children is still at considerable risk for suicide."

What else can help a suicidal patient, besides checking a list of risk factors?

During the patient's hospitalization, the patient's ideas, thoughts, and expectations with regard to suicide can be explored. Some of this might be elicited by asking patients what they imagine will happen were they to die, but deeper themes may emerge only if the interviewer reads between the lines of what a patient says out loud. For example, a common finding in depressed, suicidal patients is unresolved grief. A patient may harbor conscious or unconscious wishes to rejoin the deceased loved one. Another common thread with suicidal patients is hopelessness. This can occur when a patient believes one or more of the following:

1. I have no further options available to me.

2. No one really cares about me.

3. Everyone, including my family, would be better off without me. I am a burden to them.

4. I no longer have control over events around me.

5. Only death can offer me relief from my suffering.

During the inpatient stay, brief therapy can focus on these and similar cognitions. The distortions involved can be challenged using cognitive–behavioral techniques. For instance, if a patient is planning on acting upon the misconception that children can easily "get over" the death of a parent, the patient can be reminded gently of the reality that suicide of a parent invariably leaves considerable emotional scarring of the survivors. Dialectical behavioral approaches are useful as well. One can encourage a patient to be aware of their strong suicidal feelings, but also to recognize that those feelings do not have to be in control of the situation.

Besides more formal therapy, a suicidal crisis can also be alleviated with problem-solving and environmental manipulation related to the patient's "real life" problems, e.g., discussion about leaving a stressful job, seeking legal counsel, looking into debt consolidation, etc.

In the evaluation of a patient's suicide potential, clinicians can put some stock in their "gut feelings." This useful tool, which gets more refined with experience, is usually a reaction to the patient's level of hopelessness or a sense that the patient lacks an alliance with the treatment team. However, caution is necessary here, since gut feelings can lead the clinician astray. A dangerous situation arises when, for example, the provider identifies closely with the patient. The patient may remind the clinician of a close relative or friend, one "who would **never** commit suicide!" This identification could then lead to an underestimation of suicide risk. When a clinician feels like he or she is "really connecting" with a patient, the nature of this connection should be questioned and examined. Discussion with a colleague/supervisor is never a bad idea.

How does one assess "treatment-resistant" depression?

An inpatient psychiatric unit, especially at an academic hospital and/or at a large tertiary referral center, will invariably treat patients with "treatment-resistant" depression (TRD) (Table 2.7). This is also known as "resistant," "refractory," "treatment-refractory," or "medication-resistant" depression – among other terms [44]. A structured approach to these patients is important, given the often long and complicated history of treatment trials [45].

A common mistake in treating depression is to "diagnose" a patient as treatment resistant without looking carefully at medication adherence, which may account for up to 20% of TRD cases [46]. Non-adherence is common, greater than 50% of cases by many estimates; unsurprisingly it also leads to sooner relapse [47]. Stigma of illness may lead a patient to be non-adherent with medications. Patients may also stop medications because they feel better (and are not aware of the risk of depressive relapse), or because they simply cannot afford the medication. Reviewing pharmacy records of refills and checking blood levels of medication on admission may be useful here. Poor adherence that is unrecognized or not addressed can lead to a pattern of

Table 2.7 Correlates of treatment resistance

Inadequate trial(s)	poor adherence, side effects
	low dose(s) or short duration(s)
	drug–drug interactions
	metabolic polymorphisms
Type of depression	atypical
	psychotic
	bipolar
Co-morbidity	anxiety and/or panic
	personality traits or disorder
	alcohol and/or illicit drugs
	medical problems
Diagnostic testing	polysomnography with severe sleep disturbances
	characteristic findings on neuroimaging (controversial)
	over-activation of HPA axis
Family and environment	positive family history of mood disorder, especially in first-degree relatives
	young age of onset
	lower socioeconomic class
	non-supportive social environment
	chronic stressors
	multiple losses
	lower level of education
	occupational problems

frequent switches in medications, the "parfait sundae" layering of multiple medications in attempts to augment a partial response, and/or premature consideration of more invasive treatments such as ECT [48].

The clinician should look at possible drug–drug interactions that may have decreased the effectiveness or tolerability of past or current psychotropic agents, leading to "treatment resistance" [49, 50]. Genetically based variations in metabolism rates of various medications can lead to a history of non-responsiveness at ordinary dosages [51]. If a depressed patient is having no

Table 2.8 Medical conditions that can cause depression [27]

Tumors: either primary or metastatic to brain, especially lung cancer and pancreatic cancer; paraneoplastic syndrome

Infections: CNS syphilis, CNS HIV, meningitis; urinary tract infections, pneumonia, mononucleosis

Endocrine disorders: Cushing's syndrome, hyper/hypothyroidism, Addison's disease, hyperparathyroidism

Hematological: anemia, leukemia

Neurological: Huntington's disease, Parkinson's disease, various forms of dementia, stroke, basal ganglia degeneration, traumatic brain injury

Toxic: illicit drugs, alcohol; medication side effects

Nutrition and electrolytes: vitamin deficiencies (e.g., niacin in pellagra), hyponatremia, hypocalcemia

Other: post-myocardial infarction, renal failure, sleep apnea

response at a routine dosage of an appropriate antidepressant, and is having no side effects, a higher dose may be warranted. On the other hand, if a patient has severe side effects at low doses, further investigation into possible interactions is necessary.

Any time a reportedly treatment-resistant patient is admitted to the hospital the diagnostic picture should be carefully reexamined. This may seem obvious, especially since a clinician always needs to perform his or her own diagnostic assessment of a new patient. But TRD is a particularly frustrating problem for patients and providers alike, to the point where both sides sometimes "give up." Furthermore, confounding factors and co-morbid conditions are often missed since the depressive features are so prominent [46].

Evaluation of general medical disorders associated with depression, as listed in Table 2.8, is key. After these have been addressed or ruled out, the inpatient provider should take a step back and consider such issues as underlying personality disorders [52], severe psychosocial issues [53–56], and co-morbid Axis I disorders, especially anxiety disorders or chemical dependence [46]. In this era of psychopharmacology, many patients do not get adequate psychotherapy, and psychotherapy is the mainstay of treatment of the aforementioned conditions.

A missed diagnosis of Bipolar Disorder, either Type I or II, is a common reason for treatment resistance. Bipolar II is relatively common, and some evidence points to the presence of Bipolar II in up to 50% of depressed patients [57]. Bipolar patients demonstrate poor and/or delayed response to antidepressants [58]. When evaluating a TRD patient, one should look

Table 2.9 The rule of 3s [57]

More than	3	major depressive episodes
	3	failed marriages
	3	failed antidepressants
	3	first degree relatives with mood disorder
	3	generation family history for mood disorder
Eminence in	3	fields in the family
	3	simultaneous jobs
Proficiency in	3	languages (for US-born citizens)
	3	distinct professions (exercised simultaneously)
	3	co-morbid anxiety diagnoses
Past diagnoses of	3	personality disorders (histrionic, psychopathic, borderline)
History of	3	traits: "mood lability," "energy activity," and "daydreaming"
Flamboyance expressed in	3	bright colors
	3	substances of abuse
	3	impulse control behaviors
Simultaneous dating of	3	individuals

carefully for the presence of unrecognized symptoms – which can be subtle – of bipolar spectrum illness (Table 2.9) [57, 59]. Additional pieces of evidence might include onset of depression at a young age, a family history of Bipolar Disorder, and/or reverse neurovegetative signs [16]. Significant suspicion of bipolar spectrum illness in a TRD patient should lead the clinician towards consideration of mood-stabilizing medications rather than "unopposed" antidepressants [16, 60].

A final important consideration with treatment resistance is that hidden psychosis, accompanying a more obvious depression, can render antidepressant monotherapy ineffective [46]. The diagnosis of psychotic depression is commonly missed in a variety of psychiatric settings, including inpatient units at prestigious medical centers [61]. While it is not difficult to make the diagnosis of psychotic depression when a patient hears voices telling them they are going to die, a patient may not spontaneously bring up, for instance, the dark shadowy figures in the corners of their vision. A high index of suspicion and intensive questioning for psychotic symptoms are necessary.

What is the relationship between catatonia and severe depression?

DSM-IV-TR classifies catatonia as a sub-type of schizophrenia, and as a speci-fier for mood disorders (e.g., Major Depressive Disorder with Catatonic Fea-tures). This psychomotor syndrome can be seen in a variety of general medical, neurologic, toxic, and psychiatric conditions, including severe depression [62, 63]. Catatonic patients present with signs of motor dysregulation, which can include stupor, motor excitement, immobility, mutism, posturing, grimac-ing, stereotypy, and mannerisms (Table 2.10) [19, 64]. Some signs can be

Table 2.10 Principal features of catatonia [19]

Feature	Description
Mutism	Verbal unresponsiveness, not always associated with immobility
Stupor	Unresponsiveness, hypoactivity, and reduced or altered arousal during which the patient fails to respond to queries; when severe, the patient is mute, immobile, and does not withdraw from painful stimuli
Negativism (geganhalten)	Resistance to examiner's manipulations, whether light or vigorous, with strength equal to that applied
Posturing (catalepsy)	Maintenance of postures for long periods – including facial postures (grimacing or puckering), body postures ("psychological pillow"), or holding limbs or fingers in odd, even uncomfortable positions
Waxy flexibility	Initial resistance to induced movement followed by gradual compliance, like bending a candle
Stereotypy	Non-goal-directed, repetitive motor behavior – can also be verbal (verbigeration or palilalia)
Automatic obedience	Permission of examiner's light pressure to move limbs, despite verbal instructions to the contrary
Ambitendency	Appearing "stuck" in an indecisive, hesitant movement – elicited by offering a strong non-verbal cue (extending hand for handshake) while giving opposite verbal instruction ("Don't shake my hand")
Echophenomena	Repeating examiner's speech (echolalia) or movements (echopraxia)
Mannerisms	Odd, purposeful movements, such as holding hands as if they were handguns, saluting passersby, or exaggerating mundane movements

elicited by the examiner. For example, echopraxia is demonstrated if the clinician scratches his/her head and the patient imitates this.

A full discussion of the intricacies of catatonia is beyond the scope of this volume. However, it is important to realize that catatonic signs are easily missed on the inpatient unit. One does not have to be mute to be catatonic. This syndrome can frequently be detected in the inpatient population when the index of suspicion is high [65, 66]. When present it needs to be recognized, since specific treatments might then be indicated, including high doses of benzodiazepines, avoidance of antipsychotics (especially high-potency drugs), and possibly a referral for ECT [19, 67].

How does the inpatient clinician approach pharmacologic treatment in unipolar depression?

Clinicians should familiarize themselves with known treatment guidelines and algorithms, such as the Texas Medication Algorithm Project (TMAP) and the American Psychiatric Association (APA) Practice Guideline [68, 69]. One may also wish to be familiar with the STAR*D study [70]. While these are important resources, they are not recipes! There are simply too many random variables that crop up, including patient preferences or medication side effects, to rigidly implement a given algorithm. That said, there is evidence that algorithm-guided treatment is more effective than "treatment as usual" [71, 72].

Antidepressant psychopharmacology is a vast field that is ever changing, with dozens of medications and seemingly infinite possible combinations of medications. It would be impossible to encompass the entire literature in this modest volume. Nonetheless, combining the experience of the authors with the aforementioned algorithms and guidelines produces some useful tips with regard to various classes of medications with antidepressant action:

- The patient with new onset of depression has many choices among the various antidepressant competitors in the marketplace. The inpatient unit sees a fair share of people, young and old, who have never had medication for depression. An SSRI is the first-line choice for uncomplicated non-melancholic major depression. There has been recent debate in the literature about which SSRIs work better or are more tolerated. A meta-analysis by Gartlehner *et al.*, which supported practice guidelines by the Clinical Efficacy Assessment Subcommittee of the American College of Physicians, did not find significant differences among the SSRIs and other "second generation" antidepressants [73, 74]. However, a multiple-treatments meta-analysis performed by a group led by Cipriani showed an efficacy advantage for mirtazapine, escitalopram, venlafaxine, and sertraline [75].

- Since many inpatients have had various trials of medications or are hospitalized because of a poor response to medication, a clinician needs to be prepared to switch to a different class of antidepressant [70, 76]. Venlafaxine may be useful when SSRIs have failed, but reports of an efficacy advantage are controversial [77–79]. In the authors' experience, also demonstrated by some small studies, venlafaxine is often under-dosed [77, 80, 81]. Bupropion is another antidepressant that should be considered as a first-line monotherapy agent. It has advantages over SSRIs in its weight neutrality and lack of sexual side effects [76, 78]. Finally, mirtazapine is worth serious consideration [82]. It is very well tolerated, and some evidence suggests that it may work faster than other antidepressants [83, 84]. The sedation side effect is useful, not only in helping patients sleep, but in getting "buy in" since a patient perceives that the medication is "doing something."

- With the severity of depression seen on inpatient units, some clinicians are advocating an earlier turn to TCAs [85]. Despite known anticholinergic side effects, which can be minimized with selection of nortriptyline or desipramine, these medications can be surprisingly effective, especially with severe melancholic depression [15, 82]. Likewise, MAOIs are often not considered due to the dietary restrictions, side-effect burden, and lack of clinician familiarity [86]. But MAOIs can be quite effective, especially with atypical depression and other treatment-resistant patients [87]. There is now more complete understanding of necessary dietary precautions, leading to more options for responsible patients [88]. Keeping this option in the armamentarium is strongly recommended.

- Combinations of antidepressants are often useful, but studies of these are smaller and more complicated than those with monotherapy. Fava and Rush provide an accessible, relatively thorough overview of this area [89]. It has been found that SSRI/SNRI + bupropion can be effective and in a certain percentage of cases bupropion may also mitigate the sexual side effects of the SSRI or SNRI [89, 90]. A combination of SSRI/SNRI + mirtazapine can lead to a positive response, but the prescriber must be cautious about side effects [89]. A TCA can also be added to an SSRI when patients have had only a partial response to the SSRI [91]. Care is advised, though, with combining SSRIs and TCAs as several of the SSRIs inhibit the cytochrome P450 2D6 (CYP450 2D6) system and cause increases in the blood level of the TCA [89]. Finally, in patients with severe illness and no other options that have not been tried, an MAOI added onto TCA can be a life-saving intervention [92, 93]. This combination is fraught with *potential* hazards, though, and careful monitoring is extremely important.

- There are a number of other, non-antidepressant medications used for augmentation of a failed or partial response to an initial medication trial. Of these, the best studied is lithium augmentation [89, 94]. Lithium levels for augmentation may not need to be quite as high as for monotherapy in bipolar disorder, but an adequate trial includes levels up to 0.8 to 1.0 mEq/L. Thyroid augmentation is another useful strategy. L-triiodothronine (25–50 mcg/day) is preferred to thyroxine for augmentation [89, 94, 95]. Next, there is now a growing literature on the use of atypical antipsychotics as augmenters, and aripiprazole and quetiapine XR have received this FDA indication [96]. They may be exerting their action through an independent antidepressant effect, but also by decreasing rumination and anxiety. Caution must be exercised given the side-effect burden.

- Patients with psychotic depression (DSM-IV-TR Major Depression, Severe with Psychotic Features) are generally very ill, and require aggressive inpatient treatment. Electroconvulsive therapy provides the best response rates for these patients (see below), but if medication is the only option, patients with psychotic depression do best with a combination of an antidepressant and an antipsychotic [46, 97]. The older literature showed good response rates with the combination of perphenazine and a TCA, while the newer literature has shown similar responses with olanzapine combined with fluoxetine or sertraline [98].

What is the pharmacologic approach to *bipolar* depression on the inpatient unit?

The depressive phases of bipolar disorder are more disabling and harder to manage than the manic states. Many bipolar patients, both type I and type II, spend the majority of their illness time in a depressed state [16]. The risk of manic switch with antidepressants has been debated in the field for decades [99]. More recently, the safety, and especially the efficacy, of antidepressants in bipolar disorder, whether "unopposed" or as part of a multiple-drug regimen, has been a subject of renewed debate [58, 60]. A consensus is emerging that mood stabilizers should be the mainstay of treatment in bipolar disorder, whether the patient is currently depressed or manic [16].

At this time the FDA-approved medications for bipolar depression are the combination fluoxetine/olanzapine (start at 6/25 mg in evening, maximum of 18/75 mg/day), and quetiapine (300–600 mg/day). Lithium and lamotrigine also are effective monotherapy agents for some patients with bipolar depression. Since inpatients with bipolar depression may be admitted to the unit with "break through" depressions on seemingly adequate medication regimens, combinations of medications are often required for efficacy. Some experienced clinicians would like to see the patient fail a trial of a combination of two mood stabilizers (e.g., lithium plus lamotrigine) before proceeding to antidepressants. In the past MAOIs were popular for bipolar depression, which often has atypical features, but as mentioned above they are usually reserved for refractory cases.

When is electroconvulsive therapy considered for a psychiatric inpatient?

Patients are referred to a unit that provides ECT treatment because they have failed to achieve a response or remission with multiple, sometimes many, medication regimens. An inpatient psychiatric service that purports to treat difficult cases of depression must have an ECT program. Electroconvulsive therapy is the most effective antidepressant treatment available at this time. It should at least be "on the table" for most inpatients with depression [100]. Electroconvulsive therapy should be strongly considered for, and discussed with, patients with severe depression, especially with unrelenting suicidal thoughts or psychosis; patients with significant depression-induced medical issues (e.g., a dangerous degree of weight loss); and/or patients with co-morbid catatonic syndrome [2, 101, 102]. Electroconvulsive therapy can also be a godsend to patients with intolerable side effects. Finally, it is important to note that ECT is safe during pregnancy, safer than psychiatric medications, and is an important treatment for pregnant women with severe depression [103].

As with unipolar depressions on the inpatient unit, ECT should be considered for patients with bipolar depression. Compared to medications, ECT may have a more rapid response (often within one to two weeks) and can be especially useful in severe suicidal depressive or mixed states and situations in which nutrition and overall health are endangered [101, 102].

There are no absolute contraindications to ECT [104]. Conditions such as space-occupying brain lesions, cerebral aneurysms, arterio-venous malformations, recent myocardial infarction, and recently detached retina are viewed as complicating situations, and likely will require special consultation prior to ECT. One strong proponent of ECT has voiced the idea that "the only *absolute* contraindication to ECT is a power outage."

What are useful psychotherapeutic approaches to the depressed inpatient?

When a patient is in a deep melancholic depression, the therapeutic approach should be one of comfort, education, encouragement, and hopeful optimism. The therapy should be supportive in nature and directed at allowing the patient to express concerns and fears related to his or her illness and/or treatment. The clinician should not struggle to negate the patient's depression-tinged negative world view, even if it is delusional. However, an empathetic response to the patient's suffering can be coupled with an explanation that "that is your depression talking."

As the patient improves, the clinician may be able to do some short-term therapy directed at the major precipitants of the depression. These therapies are less likely to be useful with melancholic depressions than with the more moderate depressions. If the clinician is versed in cognitive–behavioral therapy (CBT), some of those techniques can be applied towards the patient's identified depression-generating cognitions and expectations [105–107]. Interpersonal therapy (IPT) is another form of psychotherapy that has been rigorously tested in depressed patients [108, 109]. This therapy focuses on the patient's problems with role transitions, interpersonal conflicts, role disputes, and pathological grief. If a problem in one of these four domains has been identified, the clinician can begin a process of therapy in the hospital that can be continued as an outpatient.

A specialized inpatient mood disorder program may also have therapies with CBT and IPT elements that are offered in a group therapy format. Aside from these specialized therapies, patients with all severities of depression, once stabilized, will benefit from education about the possibility of recurrences of illness and the need for close adherence to outpatient treatment.

References

1. George L, Durbin J, Sheldon T & Goering P. Patient and contextual factors related to the decision to hospitalize patients from emergency psychiatric services. *Psychiatric Services*, **53**:12 (2002), 1586–91.

2. Fink M, Abrams R, Bailine S & Jaffe R. Ambulatory electroconvulsive therapy: report of a task force of the association for convulsive therapy. Association for Convulsive Therapy. *Convulsive Therapy*, **12**:1 (1996), 42–55.

3. Jones A & Crossley D. "In the mind of another" shame and acute psychiatric inpatient care: an exploratory study. A report on phase one: service users. *Journal of Psychiatric and Mental Health Nursing*, **15**:9 (2008), 749–57.

4. Engel G. The clinical application of the biopsychosocial model. *American Journal of Psychiatry*, **137**:5 (1980), 535–44.

5. Engel G L. The need for a new medical model: a challenge for biomedicine. *Science*, **196**:4286 (1977), 129–36.

6. Mahoney J S, Palyo N, Napier G & Giordano J. The therapeutic milieu reconceptualized for the 21st century. *Archives of Psychiatric Nursing*, **23**:6 (2009), 423–9.

7. Schopp R. Depression, the insanity defense, and civil commitment: foundations in autonomy and responsibility. *International Journal of Law and Psychiatry*, **12**:1 (1989), 81.

8. Treatment Advocacy Center. State standards for assisted treatment: state by state chart. September 2008; www.treatmentadvocacycenter.org [Accessed September 23, 2009].

9. Caplan J P. Mnemonics in a mnutshell: 32 aids to psychiatric diagnosis. *Current Psychiatry*, 7:10 (2008), 27.

10. Sajatovic M & Ramirez L. *Rating Scales in Mental Health*, 2nd edn. Hudson, OH: Lexi-Comp, Inc.; 2003.

11. Maixner D. "Beyond the DSM": A lecture on descriptive psychopathology. Ann Arbor, MI; 2005.

12. Parker G. Is the diagnosis of melancholia important in shaping clinical management? *Current Opinion in Psychiatry*, **20**:3 (2007), 197–201.

13. Nelson J C & Davis J M. DST studies in psychotic depression: a meta-analysis. *American Journal of Psychiatry*, **154**:11 (1997), 1497–503.

14. Antonijevic I A. Depressive disorders – is it time to endorse different pathophysiologies? *Psychoneuroendocrinology*, **31**:1 (2006), 1–15.

15. Perry P J. Pharmacotherapy for major depression with melancholic features: relative efficacy of tricyclic versus selective serotonin reuptake inhibitor antidepressants. *Journal of Affective Disorders*, **39**:1 (1996), 1–6.

16. Thase M E. Bipolar depression: diagnostic and treatment considerations. *Development and Psychopathology*, **18**:4 (2006), 1213–30.

17. Taylor M A & Fink M. Restoring melancholia in the classification of mood disorders. *Journal of Affective Disorders*, **105**:1–3 (2008), 1–14.

18. American Psychiatric Association. Task Force on DSM-IV. *Diagnostic and Statistical Manual of Mental Disorders: DSM-IV-TR*, 4th edn. Washington, DC: American Psychiatric Association; 2000.

19. Fink M & Taylor M A. *Catatonia: A Clinician's Guide to Diagnosis and Treatment*. Cambridge, UK: Cambridge University Press; 2003.

20. Marcus S, Flynn H, Young E, Ghaziuddin N & Mudd S. Recurrent depression in women throughout the life span. In: Greden J, ed. *Review of Psychiatry. Vol. 20: Treatment of Recurrent Depression*. Washington DC: American Psychiatric Publishing, Inc.; 2001, pp. 19–58.

21. Kahn M W. Emergency psychiatry: Tools of engagement: Avoiding pitfalls in collaborating with patients. *Psychiatric Services*, **52**:12 (2001), 1571–2.

22. Bollini P, Pampallona S, Kupelnick B, Tibaldi G & Munizza C. Improving compliance in depression: a systematic review of narrative reviews. *Journal of Clinical Pharmacy and Therapeutics*, **31**:3 (2006), 253–60.

23. Blazer D G. Depression in late life: review and commentary. *Journals in Gerontology. Series A, Biological Sciences and Medical Sciences*, **58**:3 (2003), 249–65.

24. Gallo J, Rabins P, Lyketsos C, Tien A & Anthony J. Depression without sadness: functional outcomes of nondysphoric depression in later life. *Journal of the American Geriatrics Society*, **45**:5 (1997), 570.

25. Chopra M P, Sullivan J R, Feldman Z, Landes R D & Beck C. Self-, collateral- and clinician assessment of depression in persons with cognitive impairment. *Aging & Mental Health*, **12**:6 (2008), 675–83.

26. Goodwin F & Jamison K. Chapter 6. Children and adolescents. In: *Manic-Depressive Illness: Bipolar Disorders and Recurrent Depression*, 2nd edn. New York: Oxford University Press; 2007, pp. 187–221.

27. Levenson J. *Essentials of Psychosomatic Medicine*. Arlington, VA: American Psychiatric Publishing, Inc.; 2007.

28. Andreasen N C, Swayze V, 2nd, Flaum M, Alliger R & Cohen G. Ventricular abnormalities in affective disorder: clinical and demographic correlates. *American Journal of Psychiatry*, **147**:7 (1990), 893–900.

29. Herrmann L L, Le Masurier M & Ebmeier K P. White matter hyperintensities in late life depression: a systematic review. *Journal of Neurology, Neurosurgery & Psychiatry*, **79**:6 (2008), 619–24.

30. Pompili M, Innamorati M, Mann J J *et al.* Periventricular white matter hyperintensities as predictors of suicide attempts in bipolar disorders and unipolar depression. *Progress in Neuro-psychopharmacology & Biological Psychiatry*, **32**:6 (2008), 1501–7.

31. Videbech P, Ravnkilde B, Fiirgaard B *et al.* Structural brain abnormalities in unselected in-patients with major depression. *Acta Psychiatrica Scandinavica*, **103**:4 (2001), 282–6.

32. Lieberman D Z, Resnik H L & Holder-Perkins V. Environmental risk factors in hospital suicide. *Suicide & Life-threatening Behavior*, **34**:4 (2004), 448–53.

33. Busch K, Fawcett J & Jacobs D. Clinical correlates of inpatient suicide. *Journal of Clinical Psychiatry*, **64**:1 (2003), 14–19.

34. Angst J, Angst F & Stassen H H. Suicide risk in patients with major depressive disorder. *Journal of Clinical Psychiatry,* **60**:Suppl. 2 (1999), 57–62; discussion **75–76**, 113–16.

35. Burgess P, Pirkis J, Morton J & Croke E. Lessons from a comprehensive clinical audit of users of psychiatric services who committed suicide. *Psychiatric Services*, **51**:12 (2000), 1555–60.

36. Pirkis J & Burgess P. Suicide and recency of health care contacts. A systematic review. *British Journal of Psychiatry*, **173** (1998), 462–74.

37. Goodwin F K. Preventing inpatient suicide. *Journal of Clinical Psychiatry*, **64**:1 (2003), 12–13.

38. Shea S C. *The Practical Art of Suicide Assessment: A Guide for Mental Health Professionals and Substance Abuse Counselors.* New York: John Wiley; 1999.

39. Powell J, Geddes J, Hawton K, Deeks J & Goldacre M. Suicide in psychiatric hospital in-patients: Risk factors and their predictive power. *British Journal of Psychiatry*, **176**:3 (2000), 266–72.

40. Tishler C L & Reiss N S. Inpatient suicide: preventing a common sentinel event. *General Hospital Psychiatry*, **31**:2 (2009), 103–9.

41. Miller M & Hemenway D. Guns and suicide in the United States. *New England Journal of Medicine*, **359**:10 (2008), 989–91.

42. Appleby L. Suicide in psychiatric patients: risk and prevention. *British Journal of Psychiatry*, **161**:6 (1992), 749–58.

43. Malone K M, Oquendo M A, Haas G L *et al.* Protective factors against suicidal acts in major depression: reasons for living. *American Journal of Psychiatry*, **157**:7 (2000), 1084–8.

44. Berlim M T & Turecki G. What is the meaning of treatment resistant/refractory major depression (TRD)? A systematic review of current randomized trials. *European Neuropsychopharmacology*, **17**:11 (2007), 696–707.

45. Pridmore S & Turnier-Shea Y. Medication options in the treatment of treatment-resistant depression. *Australian and New Zealand Journal of Psychiatry*, **38**:4 (2004), 219–25.

46. Fagiolini A & Kupfer D J. Is treatment-resistant depression a unique subtype of depression? *Biological Psychiatry*, **53**:8 (2003), 640–8.

47. ten Doesschate M C, Bockting C L H & Schene A H. Adherence to continuation and maintenance antidepressant use in recurrent depression. *Journal of Affective Disorders*, **115**:1–2 (2009), 167–170.

48. Frye M A, Ketter T A, Leverich G S *et al.* The increasing use of polypharmacotherapy for refractory mood disorders: 22 years of study. *Journal of Clinical Psychiatry*, **61**:1 (2000), 9–15.

49. Coutts R T & Urichuk L J. Polymorphic cytochromes P450 and drugs used in psychiatry. *Cellular & Molecular Neurobiology*, **19**:3 (1999), 325–54.

50. Tanaka E & Hisawa S. Clinically significant pharmacokinetic drug interactions with psychoactive drugs: antidepressants and antipsychotics and the cytochrome P450 system. *Journal of Clinical Pharmacy & Therapeutics*, **24**:1 (1999), 7–16.

51. Vandel P, Talon J M, Haffen E & Sechter D. Pharmacogenetics and drug therapy in psychiatry – the role of the CYP2D6 polymorphism. *Current Pharmaceutical Design*, **13**:2 (2007), 241–50.

52. Thase M E. The role of Axis II comorbidity in the management of patients with treatment-resistant depression. *Psychiatric Clinics of North America*, **19**:2 (1996), 287–309.

53. Hammen C. Stress and depression. *Annual Review of Clinical Psychology*, **1**:1 (2005), 293–319.

54. Monroe S M & Reid M W. Life stress and major depression. *Current Directions in Psychological Science*, **18**:2 (2009), 68.

55. Tennant C. Life events, stress and depression: a review of recent findings. *Australian and New Zealand Journal of Psychiatry*. **36**:2 (2002), 173–82.

56. Thase M E & Howland R H. Refractory depression: relevance of psychosocial factors and therapies. *Psychiatric Annals*, **24** (1994), 232–2.

57. Akiskal H S & Akiskal H S. Searching for behavioral indicators of bipolar II in patients presenting with major depressive episodes: the "red sign," the "rule of three" and other biographic signs of temperamental extravagance, activation and hypomania. *Journal of Affective Disorders*, **84**:2–3 (2005), 279–90.

58. Ghaemi S N, Rosenquist K J, Ko J Y *et al.* Antidepressant treatment in bipolar versus unipolar depression. *American Journal of Psychiatry*, **161**:1 (2004), 163–5.

59. Thase M. Treatment-resistant depression and the bipolar spectrum: recognition and management. *Primary Psychiatry*, **13**:11 (2006), 59–67.

60. Sachs G S, Nierenberg A A, Calabrese J R *et al.* Effectiveness of adjunctive antidepressant treatment for bipolar depression. *New England Journal of Medicine*. **356**:17 (2007), 1711–22.

61. Rothschild A J, Winer J, Flint A J *et al.* Missed diagnosis of psychotic depression at 4 academic medical centers. *Journal of Clinical Psychiatry*, **69**:8 (2008), 1293–6.

62. Abrams R & Taylor M A. Catatonia. A prospective clinical study. *Archives of General Psychiatry*, **33**:5 (1976), 579–81.

63. Carroll B T, Anfinson T J, Kennedy J C *et al.* Catatonic disorder due to general medical conditions. *Journal of Neuropsychiatry & Clinical Neurosciences*, **6**:2 (1994), 122–33.

64. Joseph R. Frontal lobe psychopathology: mania, depression, confabulation, catatonia, perseveration, obsessive compulsions, and schizophrenia. *Psychiatry*. **62**:2 (1999), 138–72.

65. Rosebush P I, Hildebrand A M, Furlong B G & Mazurek M F. Catatonic syndrome in a general psychiatric inpatient population: frequency, clinical presentation, and response to lorazepam. *Journal of Clinical Psychiatry*, **51**:9 (1990), 357–62.

66. Taylor M A, Fink M. Catatonia in psychiatric classification: a home of its own. *American Journal of Psychiatry*, **160**:7 (2003), 1233–41.

67. Bush G, Fink M, Petrides G, Dowling F & Francis A. Catatonia. II. Treatment with lorazepam and electroconvulsive therapy. *Acta Psychiatrica Scandinavica*, **93**:2 (1996), 137–43.

68. American Psychiatric Association. *Practice Guideline for the Treatment of Patients with Major Depressive Disorder*, 2nd edn. Washington, DC: American Psychiatric Association; 2000.

69. Suehs B, Argo T, Bendele S *et al.* Texas Medication Algorithm Project Procedural Manual – Major Depressive Disorder Algorithms. August 6, 2008 www.dshs.state.tx.us/mhprograms/pdf/TIMA_MDD_Manual_080608.pdf [Accessed December 1, 2009].

70. Rush A J, Trivedi M H, Wisniewski S R *et al.* Acute and longer-term outcomes in depressed outpatients requiring one or several treatment steps: a STAR*D report. *American Journal of Psychiatry*, **163**:11 (2006), 1905–17.

71. Bauer M, Pfennig A, Linden M, *et al.* Efficacy of an algorithm-guided treatment compared with treatment as usual: a randomized, controlled study of inpatients with depression. *Journal of Clinical Psychopharmacology*, **29**:4 (2009), 327–33.

72. Trivedi M H, Rush A J, Crismon M L *et al.* Clinical results for patients with major depressive disorder in the Texas Medication Algorithm Project. *Archives of General Psychiatry*, **61**:7 (2004), 669–80.

73. Gartlehner G, Gaynes B N, Hansen R A *et al.* Comparative benefits and harms of second-generation antidepressants: background paper for the American College of Physicians. *Annals of Internal Medicine*, **149**:10 (2008), 734–750.

74. Qaseem A, Snow V, Denberg T D, Forciea M A & Owens D K. Using second-generation antidepressants to treat depressive disorders: a clinical practice guideline from the American College of Physicians. *Annals of Internal Medicine*, **149**:10 (2008), 725–33.

75. Cipriani A, Furukawa T A, Salanti G *et al.* Comparative efficacy and acceptability of 12 new-generation antidepressants: a multiple-treatments meta-analysis. *Lancet*, **373**:9665 (2009), 746–58.

76. Papakostas G, Fava M, Thase M. Treatment of SSRI-resistant depression: a meta-analysis comparing within-versus across-class switches. *Biological Psychiatry*, **63**:7 (2008), 699–704.

77. Nemeroff C B, Entsuah R, Benattia I *et al.* Comprehensive analysis of remission (COMPARE) with venlafaxine versus SSRIs. *Biological Psychiatry*, **63**:4 (2008), 424–34.

78. Rush A J, Trivedi M H, Wisniewski S R *et al.* Bupropion-SR, Sertraline, or Venlafaxine-XR after failure of SSRIs for depression. *New England Journal of Medicine*, **354**:12 (2006), 1231–42.

79. Weinmann S, Becker T & Koesters M. Re-evaluation of the efficacy and tolerability of venlafaxine vs SSRI: meta-analysis. *Psychopharmacology*, **196**:4 (2008), 511–20.

80. Kelsey J E. Dose–response relationship with venlafaxine. *Journal of Clinical Psychopharmacology*, **16**:3 Suppl. 2 (1996), 21S–28S.

81. Vanoli A, Lane C, Harrison C, Steen N & Young A. Adequacy of venlafaxine dose prescribing in major depression and hospital resources implications. *Journal of Psychopharmacology*, **22**:4 (2008), 434–40.

82. Fava M, Rush A, Wisniewski S *et al.* A comparison of mirtazapine and nortriptyline following two consecutive failed medication treatments for depressed outpatients: a STAR*D report. *American Journal of Psychiatry*, **163**:7 (2006), 1161.

83. Quitkin F, Taylor B & Kremer C. Does mirtazapine have a more rapid onset than SSRIs? *Journal of Clinical Psychiatry*, **62**:5 (2001), 358–61.

84. Wheatley D, Van Moffaert M, Timmerman L & Kremer C. Mirtazapine: efficacy and tolerability in comparison with fluoxetine in patients with moderate to severe major depressive disorder. *Journal of Clinical Psychiatry*, **59**:6 (1998), 306–12.

85. Gillman P K. Tricyclic antidepressant pharmacology and therapeutic drug interactions updated. *British Journal of Pharmacology*, **151**:6 (2007), 737–48.

86. Krishnan K R. Revisiting monoamine oxidase inhibitors. *Journal of Clinical Psychiatry*, **68**:Suppl. 8 (2007), 35–41.

87. McGrath P J, Stewart J W, Fava M *et al.* Tranylcypromine versus venlafaxine plus mirtazapine following three failed antidepressant medication trials for depression: a STAR*D report. *American Journal of Psychiatry*, **163**:9 (2006), 1531–41.

88. Shulman K & Walker S. A reevaluation of dietary restrictions for irreversible monoamine oxidase inhibitors. *Psychiatric Annals*, **31**:6 (2001), 378–84.

89. Fava M & Rush A. Current status of augmentation and combination treatments for major depressive disorder: a literature review and a proposal for a novel approach to improve practice. *Psychotherapy and Psychosomatics*, **75**:3 (2006), 139–53.

90. Zajecka J. Strategies for the treatment of antidepressant-related sexual dysfunction. *Journal of Clinical Psychiatry*, **62**:Suppl. 3 (2001), 35–43.

91. Nelson J C, Mazure C M, Jatlow P I, Bowers M B, Jr. & Price L H. Combining norepinephrine and serotonin reuptake inhibition mechanisms for treatment of depression: a double-blind, randomized study. *Biological Psychiatry*, **55**:3 (2004), 296–300.

92. Goldberg R S & Thornton W E. Combined tricyclic–MAOI therapy for refractory depression: a review, with guidelines for appropriate usage. *Journal of Clinical Pharmacology*, **18**:2–3 (1978), 143–7.

93. White K & Simpson G. Combined MAOI-tricyclic antidepressant treatment: a reevaluation. *Journal of Clinical Psychopharmacology*, **1**:5 (1981), 264–82.

94. Nierenberg A A, Fava M, Trivedi M H *et al.* A comparison of lithium and T3 augmentation following two failed medication treatments for depression: a STAR*D report. *American Journal of Psychiatry*, **163**:9 (2006), 1519–30.

95. Kelly T F & Lieberman D Z. Long term augmentation with T3 in refractory major depression. *Journal of Affective Disorders*, **115**:1–2 (2009), 230–3.

96. Nelson J C & Papakostas G I. Atypical antipsychotic augmentation in major depressive disorder: a meta-analysis of placebo-controlled randomized trials. *American Journal of Psychiatry*, **166**:9 (2009), 980–91.

97. Birkenhager T K, Pluijms E M & Lucius S A P. ECT response in delusional versus non-delusional depressed inpatients. *Journal of Affective Disorders*, **74**:2 (2003), 191–5.

98. Meyers B S, Flint A J, Rothschild A J *et al.* A double-blind randomized controlled trial of olanzapine plus sertraline vs olanzapine plus placebo for psychotic depression: the study of pharmacotherapy of psychotic depression (STOP-PD). *Archives of General Psychiatry*, **66**:8 (2009), 838–47.

99. Bunney W, Jr, Murphy D, Goodwin F & Borge G. The switch process from depression to mania: relationship to drugs which alter brain amines. *Lancet*, **1**:655 (1970), 1022–7.

100. Maixner D & Taylor M. Section I – The efficacy and safety of electroconvulsive therapy. In: Tyrer P & Silk K, eds. *Cambridge Textbook of Effective Treatments in Psychiatry.* Cambridge: Cambridge University Press; 2008.

101. American Psychiatric Association, Committee on Electroconvulsive Therapy, Weiner R D. *The Practice of Electroconvulsive Therapy: Recommendations for Treatment, Training, and Privileging: A Task Force Report of the American Psychiatric Association*, 2nd edn. Washington, DC: American Psychiatric Association; 2001.

102. Scott A. *The ECT Handbook*. London: Royal College of Psychiatrists; 2005, pp. 1–243.

103. Anderson E L & Reti I M. ECT in pregnancy: a review of the literature from 1941 to 2007. *Psychosomatic Medicine*, **71**:2 (2009), 235–42.

104. Kelly K & Zisselman M. Update on electroconvulsive therapy (ECT) in older adults. *Journal of the American Geriatrics Society*, **48**:5 (2000), 560–6.

105. Beck A. *Cognitive Therapy and the Emotional Disorders*. New York: International University Press; 1976.

106. Durrant C, Clarke I, Tolland A *et al.* Designing a CBT service for an acute inpatient setting: a pilot evaluation study. *Clinical Psychology and Psychotherapy*, **14**:2 (2007), 117.

107. Stuart S, Wright J, Thase M & Beck A. Cognitive therapy with inpatients. *General Hospital Psychiatry*, **19**:1 (1997), 42–50.

108. Elkin I. The NIMH treatment of depression collaborative research program: where we began and where we are. In: Bergin A & Garfield S, eds. *Handbook of Psychotherapy and Behaviour Change.* New York: Wiley; 1994.

109. Schramm E, van Calker D, Dykierek P *et al.* An intensive treatment program of interpersonal psychotherapy plus pharmacotherapy for depressed inpatients: acute and long-term results. *American Journal of Psychiatry*, **164**:5 (2007), 768–77.

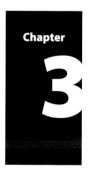

The inpatient with mania

When specific diagnoses are mentioned, we are referring to diagnoses and criteria as listed in the *Diagnostic and Statistical Manual of Mental Disorders*, 4th edition, text revision (DSM-IV-TR) unless otherwise specified.

What are the issues with acute manic and mixed-manic states on the inpatient unit?

Most inpatient clinicians have little problem recognizing classic mania, as it presents with a familiar complex of signs and symptoms: elation, expansiveness, rapid speech with flight of ideas, grandiosity, spending sprees, and hypersexuality [1]. A manic episode differs from a psychotic break in schizophrenia since a manic patient will exhibit people-seeking behavior as well as an overall quality of over-activation (Table 3.1). However, this pattern of acute euphoric mania may be less common than in the past. Increasingly, patients require hospitalization for manic symptoms combined with irritability, suicidal preoccupations, and dysphoric mood. This is the so-called "mixed state," which, depending on one's definition, 40% of bipolar patients will experience at some point in their clinical course [2]. The most conservative criteria (i.e., for DSM-IV-TR Bipolar I, Current Episode Mixed) state that patients must simultaneously meet full criteria for both a manic episode and a major depressive episode. However, in clinical practice it is more common, and some argue more useful, to apply more inclusive criteria (Table 3.2) [3, 4]. The increasing representation of such patients on inpatient units may be the result of an increased threshold of dangerousness for admission to hospitals – that is, euphoric manic patients can sometimes be managed in an outpatient setting, while the more lethal mixed-state patients will require hospitalization. It has also been speculated that the increased frequency of mixed states is related to common use of antidepressants in both diagnosed and undiagnosed bipolar patients [5].

Mixed states can be conceptualized using Kraepelin's triad of affect that includes volition (physical activity), emotion (ranging from dysphoria to euphoria), and intellect (rate or process of thoughts) (Figure 3.1) [6, 7]. In

Table 3.1 *In our experience...* How to recognize the manic patient at first encounter

Overly friendly, asks intrusive questions, comments on the clinician's appearance

Trouble conforming to the structure of an interview

Asks to get up frequently to go to the bathroom, get a drink of water, etc.

Lots of drawings, journal writings, magazine/newspaper clippings, or detailed diagrams taped to the wall or in disorganized stacks in room

Very difficult to interrupt, and will not be able to sustain listening to the clinician

Bragging about famous people they know, or their own talents

May break into song in the middle of a sentence, use lots of puns or clever language

Can turn quickly from elated to irritable, especially when thwarted

Remember: You may find manic patients entertaining – until you frustrate them

Table 3.2 The "Cincinnati" criteria for mixed mania

Full manic or hypomanic episode

AND three or more of the following depressive symptoms:

> Depressed mood
>
> Diminished interest or pleasure in all or nearly all activities
>
> Substantial weight gain or increase in appetite
>
> Hypersomnia
>
> Psychomotor retardation
>
> Fatigue or loss of energy
>
> Feelings of worthlessness or excessive/inappropriate guilt
>
> Feelings of helplessness or hopelessness
>
> Recurrent thoughts of death, suicide, and/or suicide plan; and/or a suicide attempt

Depressive symptoms **NOT** counted (i.e., that could also be due to mania):

> Insomnia
>
> Reduced appetite
>
> Psychomotor agitation
>
> Diminished ability to concentrate

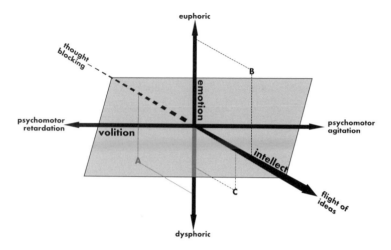

Figure 3.1 3-D model of Kraepelinian Mood States – "A" represents melancholic depression, "B" represents euphoric mania, and "C" represents a mixed state.

the Kraepelinian tradition, mixed bipolar states consist of physical agitation, dysphoria, and racing thoughts. This combination puts mixed-state patients at heightened risk for suicide. Consequently, patients with acute mixed bipolar states bear extra close monitoring on the inpatient unit [4].

Though historically, psychiatric nosologists have made much of the distinction between schizophrenia and bipolar disorder, there are instances where the patient's presentation does not lend itself to easy categorization. Some patients are manic but have mood-incongruent psychotic symptoms that lead to a misdiagnosis of schizophrenia. The diagnosis of schizoaffective disorder is often erroneously evoked to describe mixtures of mood-incongruent delusions and mood symptoms. This diagnosis should be reserved for those patients who show psychotic symptoms in the absence of mood symptoms as described in DSM-IV-TR.

What circumstances lead to the hospitalization of a patient with acute mania?

Manic and mixed-state patients are often admitted through the emergency department in highly agitated states in which they pose a danger of acting out violently toward themselves or others (Table 3.3). These patients frequently lack insight into the need for treatment, and are likely to require involuntary admission. Good documentation of the dangerousness is key. Euphorically manic patients with behaviors that are out of control but not dangerous, like profligate spending behavior or promiscuous sexual conduct, are also

Table 3.3 Reasons to hospitalize a patient with mania

High degree of desperation or hopelessness (especially common with mixed states)

Serious suicide attempt or ideation, or history of suicide attempt in a similar mood state

Recent violence or history of violence in a similar mood state

Involvement in actions that are dangerous or can ruin a patient's reputation or credit

Unreliable or absent support system

High probability of rapid deterioration without intensive and aggressive treatment

Accompanying psychosis

Medical issues that complicate aggressive pharmacologic treatment

candidates for admission. But, involuntary commitment may be difficult, depending on the laws and precedent in the specific jurisdiction. Since denial of illness and impaired insight are hallmarks of mania, hospitalization of patients who are not overtly dangerous is often delayed – either until something happens that demonstrates to the patient that he/she needs help (e.g., a family conflict or being arrested) or until the patient displays riskier behavior.

What is the approach to the acutely manic patient on the inpatient unit?

The assessment of the acute manic patient begins with the history [8]. Information from an ancillary source is always useful, and especially so when the patient is so disorganized that obtaining accurate history from the patient is unlikely. Many manic patients, even those without psychotic features, have such limited insight into their behaviors that their families are the most reliable sources of historical information, with the caveat that family members can give inaccurate information, too [9]. Once a patient hits the psychotic manic stage, differentiation from schizophrenia can be difficult with the interview alone. History obtained from a spouse or parent that outlines a progression from hypomanic gregariousness and heightened energy to a fulminate psychotic, manic state can aid in this distinction. Furthermore, family members may have observed depressive periods in the patient's life that suggest the presence of the mood cycling of bipolar disorder.

A positive family history of bipolar disorder can be a critical factor in diagnosis of the psychotic/manic inpatient. Although mapping the exact loci of the genome associated with genetic transmission of bipolar disorder is a work in progress, a strong genetic contribution to bipolar disorder is demonstrated by the concordance rate of 80% in monozygotic twins for Bipolar I disorder [10].

Often a manic patient is too disorganized to present accurate historical information during the evaluation interview. However, assessment of the patient's mental state does not necessarily require full co-operation from the patient. Observation of the patient in the interview setting and careful documentation of the mental status can bring the clinician considerably close to a definitive diagnosis of mania. Writing down verbatim quotes from the patient, which can be difficult with quick, tangential speech, allows flight of ideas or other forms of thought disorder to be seen more readily. These snippets are also useful if a case for hospitalization needs to be made to an insurance reviewer or in court.

Some clinicians find it helpful to utilize a more formal, objective rating scale to document the severity of the mania upon admission and to chart progress throughout the hospitalization. One popular scale is the Young Mania Rating Scale (YMRS) [11], a clinician-rated instrument that has been used in many studies of bipolar medication efficacy. The history, obtained by piecing together the written record, ancillary information from family and other sources, and the patient's own account of illness; the mental status examination; and a rating scale – all combined – will go a long way toward confirming the diagnosis of mania and of bipolar disorder in general.

In the instance of a patient with bipolar disorder hospitalized with an episode of mania, one task is to ask "why now?" Patients will decompensate into mania for a variety of reasons, including poor adherence to medication, drug–drug interactions leading to inadequate blood levels of mood stabilizers, major life stressors, medical illness, disruptions in sleep/wake cycle, and use of substances [12, 13]. Some very compliant patients may just "break through" an adequate medication regimen due to the natural progression and cyclical nature of the illness.

Patients with manic symptoms should be carefully examined for the presence of co-morbid conditions. Substance use is very common in bipolar disorder, with a lifetime co-occurrence frequency of 50 to 60% [10]. In addition, drugs such as amphetamine [14] or cocaine [15] can simulate a manic episode in a patient who does not have bipolar disorder. Cannabis use has been implicated as a risk factor for psychosis [16]. Because patients are not always forthcoming about their substance use, a drug screen should be part of the initial assessment of the manic patient.

Manic states can arise from other medical illnesses, *especially* in older patients [17]. This situation is sometimes referred to as "secondary mania" or "organic mood disorder," and in current DSM-IV-TR terminology as Mood Disorder Due to a General Medical Condition. Aside from neurological disease (see below), endocrine issues such as hyperthyroidism [18] and exogenous steroid treatment [19], as well as infections [20, 21], have been implicated. Assessment of electrolytes, liver function, and thyroid function, as well as blood counts and a urinalysis to screen for infection, are important. Baseline liver and renal function is necessary before starting many of the medications used to treat the manic patient anyway.

Neurological etiologies deserve special attention, given the frequent over-lap between neurological disease and psychiatric symptoms. Mania can arise from traumatic brain injury [22, 23], stroke [24], epilepsy [25], and multiple sclerosis [26], among other causes [17]. The need for imaging studies is deter-mined by the clinical picture. New onset mania in an older patient with a reliable history of no previous mood disorder should prompt consideration of a brain scan. Moreover, significant cognitive impairment or focal neuro-logical signs in manic patients of *any* age should be investigated with imaging as well. When they are identifiable, lesions are often in the right hemisphere and either orbitofrontal or basotemporal [27].

Some form of personality testing may be useful during the hospitalization of the manic patient, but will be more accurate and meaningful if completed toward the end of the patient's stay. (One of the controversial areas in psy-chiatry is the relation of bipolar disorder to borderline personality disorder [7]; experts in personality disorder and those in mood disorders line up with their allegiance to one or the other diagnosis when confronted with a puzzling patient.) Some clinicians find that an objective measure of personality is at least useful in outlining and documenting the patient's temperament, strengths, and vulnerabilities as a prelude to what will likely be lifelong treat-ment. In addition, neuropsychological testing can be useful in delineating the bipolar patient's pattern of cognitive deficits, which can be demonstrated even with bipolar patients in remission [28].

What are the first priorities in managing the patient with acute mania?

The initial goals in managing acute mania in the inpatient setting are to settle the patient and to begin to restore regular sleep patterns. Close attention must be paid to the safety of the manic patient, the other patients, and the staff; as well as the impact of the patient's state on the milieu. Sometimes one agitated patient snowballs into ten agitated patients. Manic patients can be volatile, paranoid, enraged, and/or combative. As the commonly used mood stabilizers such as lithium and valproate do not work immediately, clinicians on inpatient units need to develop expertise in the management of acute agitation [29, 30].

Early identification of agitation and pre-emptive medication interventions will decrease the time spent in seclusion/restraints; likely even eliminating the need for these drastic measures altogether. As discussed in Chapter 1, some inpatient units have developed treatment protocols that utilize some measure of agitation, such as the Behavioral Activity Rating Scale (BARS) [31] or the Positive and Negative Syndrome Scale (PANSS) [32] to trigger a medication algorithm based on the level of agitation (Table 3.4).

There is really no difference between the pharmacologic management of an acutely agitated manic patient and the treatment of patients with agitation due

Table 3.4 Behavioral Activity Rating Scale (BARS) [31]

1	difficult or unable to arouse
2	asleep but responds normally to verbal or physical contact
3	drowsy, appears sedated
4	quiet and awake (normal level of activity)
5	signs of overt activity, calms down with instructions
6	extremely or continuously active, not requiring restraint
7	violent, requires restraint

to paranoid psychoses in schizophrenia (see Figure 1.3). When patients are willing to take oral medications, choices include risperidone oral or orally disintegrating tablet (ODT) (Risperdal M-Tab) 1 to 2 mg, olanzapine oral or ODT (Zyprexa Zydis) 5 to 10 mg, aripiprazole oral or ODT (Abilify Discmelt) 10 mg, or lorazepam oral 1 to 2 mg. There is no difference in time of onset of action between the "normal" oral formulation and the ODT – the dissolving tablets dissolve and the resulting solution is swallowed and absorbed in the gastrointestinal (GI) tract [33–36]. Many agitated manic patients will be in the hospital on involuntary status, and many of those will be unwilling to take oral medication. First-line medication choices for this group include ziprasidone 20 mg intramuscular (IM) (may repeat in 4 hrs, limit of 40 mg per 24-hr period); aripiprazole 9.75 mg IM (may repeat after 2 hrs if necessary); olanzapine 10 mg IM (may repeat in 2 hrs, limit of 30 mg per 24-hr period); and haloperidol 5 to 10 mg IM every 2 to 4 hrs as necessary. Each of these can be combined with lorazepam 1 to 2 mg IM for added sedative effect. (Although the manufacturers of olanzapine recommend against combined use of IM lorazepam and olanzapine due to risk of respiratory depression [33], there is not an absolute contraindication. However, close monitoring of patients' respiratory status is necessary.) Some clinicians add benztropine 1 mg IM when using IM haloperidol, especially in younger muscular men who are more prone to extra-pyramidal symptoms (EPS).

Non-pharmacologic measures – such as re-direction, limit-setting, verbal interventions, and one-to-one nursing care – can be effective alone with mildly agitated patients, but with moderate or severe agitation they are generally a supplement to pharmacologic interventions [30, 37]. (The dementia literature is rich with examples that are often applicable to non-demented patients [38].) Seclusion or restraints should be considered last resorts, only to be employed when patients have acted out in a violent way and are thought to be an imminent danger of repeating their violent actions, or when a patient is not responsive to even high-dose pharmacologic treatment [39].

Normalization of the sleep/wake cycle is an important goal with manic patients [40, 41]. Although sleep may not fully return to normal until the mood is well stabilized, most patients will suffer less distress if provided relief of insomnia. A medication already prescribed for the patient, i.e., the atypical antipsychotic and/or benzodiazepine, can be given mostly (or all) at night. Alternatively, a short-acting hypnotic agent such as zolpidem or temazepam can be added to the patient's regimen.

What longer term medication strategies are used for bipolar mania?

There have been a number of algorithms and guidelines published – such as the Texas Implementation of Medication Algorithm [42], the Expert Consensus Guidelines [43], the British Association for Psychopharmacology Guidelines [44], and the American Psychiatric Association Practice Guideline for Treatment of Patients with Bipolar Disorder [45], to assist the clinician in the systematic treatment of mania in bipolar disorders. Individual patients, however, present unique problems and these guidelines need to be applied in a flexible fashion. Furthermore, clinicians should note that the recommendations contained in these guidelines may shift over time and that guidelines differ from each other in certain respects. (A 2005 paper by Fountoulakis and colleagues provides a broad overview of various guidelines, including differences between them [46].)

Willing patients with *newly* diagnosed bipolar disorder should be started on lithium or valproate as soon as possible, in addition to medications prescribed for agitation as discussed above [47, 48]. While response will take several days, these medications will be the mainstay of ongoing therapy. Early introduction allows for assessment and treatment of side effects, and also gets the patient in the habit of taking the medication. Administering one of these mood stabilizers from the beginning may also allow earlier decrease in dosage or discontinuation of the benzodiazepine and atypical antipsychotic (Table 3.5).

More recently than most of the above guidelines were developed, several atypical antipsychotics have been studied and approved as monotherapy alternatives to lithium and valproate [48]. In addition, many clinicians will use these agents as adjuncts to lithium or valproate in cases of severe mania, even if the patient is not agitated.

Lithium is the "benchmark" bipolar medication – for good reason [49]. It is effective for mania and has prophylactic action against the depressive pole of bipolar illness. It is the only mood stabilizer that has an "anti-suicide" effect [49, 50]. There are also data suggesting that lithium has neuroprotective and neurotrophic effects [51, 52]. Most patients will be able to tolerate a starting dose of 300 mg twice daily, but this should be reduced considerably in the elderly or in patients who are skittish about side effects. Some clinicians use more aggressive initial lithium dosing, up to 1200 mg daily, or lithium loading strategies [53, 54]. These are only appropriate in healthy young patients with

Table 3.5 Pharmacologic agents used for mania

Medication/starting dose	Comments
Lithium: 150 to 300 mg twice a day	used for acute mania for over 50 years
	monotherapy or as part of combination for severe mania
	narrow therapeutic index
	drug interactions include non-steroidal anti-inflammatory drugs, antihypertensives
Valproate: 250 mg three times a day; or loading dose 20 mg/kg	may work faster than lithium, especially if loaded
	may be better than lithium for mixed states
	available as extended release as well
Carbamazepine: 200 mg twice a day; **Oxcarbazepine**: 300 mg twice day	second-line, consider for obese patients
	less evidence for oxcarbazepine, may have fewer side effects.
Topiramate: 25 mg twice a day	third-line, usually as part of a combination
	very sedating
	weight neutral or even some weight loss
Atypical antipsychotics	majority have been approved for acute mania
	also used in combination with lithium or valproate
	clozapine for the most refractory inpatients
	baseline lipid profile/fasting glucose needed
Typical (traditional) antipsychotics	largely supplanted by atypicals
	may still be considered in refractory mania
Benzodiazepines	useful adjuncts for agitation and insomnia
	not really "anti-manic" alone

no cardiac or renal disease. They can tolerate the dosing regimen well, but might have gastrointestinal side effects, tremor, or weakness. Close monitoring of trough blood levels of lithium is standard on the inpatient unit. Severe mania may require a blood level as high as 1.0 to 1.2 mEq/L.

Valproate may be preferable over lithium for mixed states and mania with associated substance use disorders, but does not appear to confer any advantage in rapid-cycling patients [46, 55]. Some patients can tolerate an initial dose of 20 mg/kg (1000–2500 mg), in divided doses, but other patients have significant GI upset with this dosing [56]. An alternative is to start with 250 mg three times per day, obtain a trough blood level after two days, then adjust accordingly. The GI side effects can be decreased with ranitidine 150 mg twice daily.

The more challenging manic patients are those who are already taking one or more mood stabilizers but are manic nonetheless. Polypharmacy is often necessary here, but attention must be given to potential drug interactions. Lithium is relatively safe in combination with other medications, as long as drug levels are monitored closely. However, there have been a few case reports of severe adverse effects resulting from the combination of lithium and carbamazepine, regardless of level of either drug [57]. Furthermore, combining valproate and carbamazepine can lead to build up of an active metabolite of carbamazepine, 10,11-epoxide, which is not detected in routine assays of carbamazepine. Also, valproate displaces carbamazepine from protein-binding sites, increasing free carbamazepine levels [58]. Therefore one needs to reduce the carbamazepine dose by 40 to 50% when combining the two agents. Carbamazepine is a useful anti-manic agent, and unlike valproate and lithium it is relatively weight neutral, but it is relegated to second-tier status because of these sorts of drug interactions. Since the clinical utility of measurement of various total and free-drug levels is still unclear, close clinical observation is a strict requirement in these complex situations [58–61].

Some patients are not responsive to, or intolerant of, the commonly used medications mentioned thus far. In such cases the provider needs to consider use of first-generation antipsychotics and/or "third-line" agents such as oxcarbazepine or topiramate, for which there are as yet few controlled studies [43, 44, 47]. Clozapine is a "last resort" medication for mania, not because of lack of efficacy but rather due to its potential for causing severe weight gain and the ongoing need for monitoring of the complete blood count (CBC) [62]. Infrequently, a patient with treatment-resistant mania may require electroconvulsive therapy (ECT) [63]. It is especially important to consider ECT for those patients who present with the syndrome described as "delirious mania," a severe form of illness with some semblance to catatonic excitement [64].

What psychological issues are associated with treatment of bipolar disorder?

Experienced clinicians have observed that many patients with bipolar disorder have trouble recognizing emotional states in themselves and in others [65]. This deficit in self-awareness in evidenced by patients' lack of detection or acknowledgment of developing manic states, even though early intervention could potentially avoid the need for hospitalization. There is a great need for patient education about warning signs of illness. Bipolar patients as a group also show mood-*independent* character traits of increased impulsivity, decreased conscientiousness, and a diluted sense of duty and responsibility [66]. Studies of co-morbidity of personality disorders with bipolar disorder utilizing DSM criteria show that bipolar patients are three times more likely than a control group to have one or more personality disorders [67], with the most frequent being obsessive–compulsive (17%), narcissistic (8%), and borderline (7%) personality disorders [68]. When bipolar disorder is accompanied by personality pathology, it will almost certainly complicate the therapeutic alliance between the clinician and the bipolar patient on the inpatient unit, and the clinician will need to adjust the therapeutic approach accordingly.

Despite this association of bipolarity with personality disorders, other research has found that creativity, especially in the artistic realm, is over-represented in the bipolar population and in their offspring [69, 70]. Bipolar patients who pride themselves on their creative abilities may see treatment as dampening their artistic productivity. The authors have had some success in these instances with reminders to the patient that episodes of untreated illness and frequent hospitalizations for acute mania detract from lifetime creative output to a greater degree than being "just normal" ever will [71]. A related dynamic that affects adherence to medication is the addictive nature of mania itself. It may take several hospitalizations before a patient finally decides that it is worth it to give up the cocaine-like euphoria of mania in exchange for "boring" stability.

A patient with a long history of bipolar disorder bargained with his psychiatrist to maintain him at a lithium level of 0.2 to 0.3 mEq/L. He thought that this sub-therapeutic level would give him some protection against severe mania but still allow the hypomanic periods that he had come to relish. Unfortunately, this calibration did not provide adequate prophylaxis and the patient ended up hospitalized with acute mania. As he came down from his manic state, all the various inpatient staff members – psychiatrist, social worker, activities therapist, and nursing staff – directed their efforts toward helping the patient examine his attitude about medication, the quality of his life without manic highs, and his level of support from family. He finally decided to allow a higher, more protective, lithium level.

What non-pharmacologic treatment helps the manic patient on the inpatient unit?

Once acute mania has resolved with treatment in the hospital, patients may become more amenable to an exploration of the stressors that led to a relapse

Table 3.6 *In our experience*. . . Dealing with a manic patient on the inpatient unit

Avoid arguing with an acutely manic patient. It is futile to confront his/her denial of illness early in the admission. Short, focused interviews work best.

Use whatever means necessary to help the patient get a good night of sleep.

Be prepared for a post-manic depression with significant shame and guilt about what the patient did while manic.

As the patient stabilizes, give him/her some good readings about the illness, including biographies of successfully treated bipolar patients.

Emphasize the patient's ownership of the illness and the need for self-management after discharge.

Offer the patient a lot of reassurance.

Help staff set appropriate limits and avoid over-stimulation of patient.

Remember: Don't feel guilty about "taking away" the patient's mania. . . it destroys careers, relationships, and lives

(Table 3.6). Patients who have relapsed due to poor medication adherence can be reeducated about the chronic and recurrent nature of bipolar disorder – how it is an illness that is managed, not cured. In addition, as patients "come down" from mania and survey the detritus of their manic state, they may experience feelings of shame and demoralization and will be in need of supportive therapy. Daily suicide-risk assessment is important at this vulnerable stage of illness. Groups and activities on the unit, especially if they are specifically targeted toward mood disorder patients, offer a forum for ventilation and support. Contact with family, including family sessions with the patient present, can help to identify the stressors facing the patient and can ease the reentry into life outside the hospital. A high-quality inpatient program for patients with bipolar disorders will incorporate a focus on bipolar disease management and self-care skills [72, 73], and will include preparation for the transition to services in the outpatient sector.

References

1. Sadock B J, Sadock V A & Kaplan H I. *Kaplan & Sadock's Comprehensive Textbook of Psychiatry*, 8th edn. Philadelphia, PA: Lippincott Williams & Wilkins; 2004.

2. Akiskal H, Hantouche E, Bourgeois M *et al.* Gender, temperament, and the clinical picture in dysphoric mixed mania: findings from a French national study (EPIMAN). *Journal of Affective Disorders*, **50**:2–3 (1998), 175–86.

3. McElroy S, Keck P, Jr, Pope H, Jr, *et al.* Clinical and research implications of the diagnosis of dysphoric or mixed mania or hypomania. *American Journal of Psychiatry*, **149**:12 (1992), 1633.

4. Sato T, Bottlender R, Tanabe A & Möller H. Cincinnati criteria for mixed mania and suicidality in patients with acute mania. *Comprehensive Psychiatry*, **45**:1 (2004), 62–9.

5. Koukopoulos A. Agitated depression as a mixed state and the problem of melancholia. *Psychiatric Clinics of North America*, **22**:3 (1999), 547–64.

6. Marneros A. Origin and development of concepts of bipolar mixed states. *Journal of Affective Disorders*, **67**:1–3 (2001), 229–40.

7. MacKinnon D & Pies R. Affective instability as rapid cycling: theoretical and clinical implications for borderline personality and bipolar spectrum disorders. *Bipolar Disorders*, **8**:1 (2006), 1.

8. MacKinnon R A, Michels R & Buckley P J. *The Psychiatric Interview in Clinical Practice*, 2nd edn. Washington, DC: American Psychiatric Publishing; 2006.

9. Roy M A, Walsh D & Kendler K S. Accuracies and inaccuracies of the family history method: a multivariate approach. *Acta Psychiatrica Scandinavica*, **93**:4 (1996), 224–34.

10. Goodwin F & Jamison K. *Manic-depressive Illness: Bipolar Disorders and Recurrent Depression*. USA: Oxford University Press; 2007.

11. Young R, Biggs J, Ziegler V & Meyer D. A rating scale for mania: reliability, validity and sensitivity. *British Journal of Psychiatry,* **133:5** (1978), 429.

12. Ellicott A, Hammen C, Gitlin M, Brown G & Jamison K. Life events and the course of bipolar disorder. *American Journal of Psychiatry*, **147**:9 (1990), 1194.

13. Gitlin M, Swendsen J, Heller T & Hammen C. Relapse and impairment in bipolar disorder. *American Journal of Psychiatry*, **152**:11 (1995), 1635.

14. Lineberry T W & Bostwick M J. Methamphetamine abuse: a perfect storm of complications. *Mayo Clinic Proceedings*, **81**:1 (2006), 77–84.

15. Siqueland L, Horn A, Moras K *et al.* Cocaine-induced mood disorder: prevalence rates and psychiatric symptoms in an outpatient cocaine-dependent sample. *American Journal on Addictions*, **8**:2 (1999), 165–9.

16. Arseneault L, Cannon M, Witton J & Murray R M. Causal association between cannabis and psychosis: examination of the evidence. *Focus*, **5**:2 (2007), 270–8.

17. Van Gerpen M, Johnson J & Winstead D. Mania in the geriatric patient population: a review of the literature. *American Journal of Geriatric Psychiatry*, 7:3 (1999), 188.

18. Lee S, Chow C, Wing Y *et al.* Mania secondary to thyrotoxicosis. *British Journal of Psychiatry*, **159** (1991), 712–13.

19. Sirois F. Steroid psychosis: a review. *General Hospital Psychiatry*, **25**:1 (2003), 27–33.

20. Maurizi C. Influenza and mania: a possible connection with the locus ceruleus. *Southern Medical Journal*, **78**:2 (1985), 207.

21. Schwartz R. Manic psychosis in connection with Q-fever. *British Journal of Psychiatry*, **124**:579 (1974), 140.

22. Jorge R, Robinson R, Starkstein S *et al.* Secondary mania following traumatic brain injury. *American Journal of Psychiatry*, **150**:6 (1993), 916.

23. Shukla S, Cook B, Mukherjee S, Godwin C & Miller M. Mania following head trauma. *American Journal of Psychiatry*, **144**:1 (1987), 93.

24. Cummings J & Mendez M. Secondary mania with focal cerebrovascular lesions. *American Journal of Psychiatry*, **141**:9 (1984), 1084.

25. Lyketsos C, Stoline A, Longstreet P *et al.* Mania in temporal lobe epilepsy. *Cognitive and Behavioral Neurology*, **6**:1 (1993), 19.

26. Diaz-Olavarrieta C, Cummings J, Velazquez J & Garcia de al Cadena C. Neuropsychiatric manifestations of multiple sclerosis. *Journal of Neuropsychiatry and Clinical Neurosciences*, **11**:1 (1999), 51.

27. Shulman K. Disinhibition syndromes, secondary mania and bipolar disorder in old age. *Journal of Affective Disorders*, **46**:3 (1997), 175–82.

28. Quraishi S & Frangou S. Neuropsychology of bipolar disorder: a review. *Journal of Affective Disorders*, **72**:3 (2002), 209–26.

29. Battaglia J. Pharmacological management of acute agitation. *Drugs*, **65**:9 (2005), 1207–22.

30. Citrome L. Agitation III: Pharmacologic treatment of agitation. In: Glick R L, Berlin J S, Fishkind A B & Zeller S L eds. *Emergency Psychiatry: Principles and Practice.* Philadelphia: Wolters Kluwer Health/Lippincott Williams & Wilkins; 2008.

31. Swift R H, Harrigan E P, Cappelleri J C, Kramer D & Chandler L P. Validation of the behavioural activity rating scale (BARS): a novel measure of activity in agitated patients. *Journal of Psychiatric Research*, **36**:2 (2002), 87–95.

32. Kay S R, Fiszbein A & Opler L A. The positive and negative syndrome scale (PANSS) for schizophrenia. *Schizophrenia Bulletin*, **13**:2 (1987), 261–76.

33. Zyprexa [package insert]. Indianapolis, IN: Eli Lilly and Company; 2009.

34. Risperdal [package insert]. Titusville, NJ: Ortho-McNeil-Janssen Pharmaceuticals, Inc.; 2009.

35. Abilify [package insert]. Tokyo: Otsuka Pharmaceutical Co, Ltd.; 2009.

36. Markowitz J, DeVane C, Malcolm R *et al.* Pharmacokinetics of olanzapine after single-dose oral administration of standard tablet versus normal and sublingual administration of an orally disintegrating tablet in normal volunteers. *Journal of Clinical Pharmacology*, **46**:2 (2006), 164.

37. Novitsky M Jr, Julius R & Dubin W. Non-pharmacologic management of violence in psychiatric emergencies. *Primary Psychiatry*, **16**:9 (2009), 49–53.

38. Teri L, Logsdon R & McCurry S. Nonpharmacologic treatment of behavioral disturbance in dementia. *Medical Clinics of North America*, **86**:3 (2002), 641–56.

39. Donat D. Encouraging alternatives to seclusion, restraint, and reliance on PRN drugs in a public psychiatric hospital. *Psychiatric Services*, **56**:9 (2005), 1105.

40. Bauer M, Grof P, Rasgon N *et al.* Temporal relation between sleep and mood in patients with bipolar disorder. *Bipolar Disorders*, **8**:2 (2006), 160.

41. Harvey A. Sleep and circadian rhythms in bipolar disorder: seeking synchrony, harmony, and regulation. *American Journal of Psychiatry*, **165**:7 (2008), 820.

42. Suppes T, Dennehy E B, Hirschfeld R M A *et al.* The Texas implementation of medication algorithms: update to the algorithms for treatment of bipolar I disorder. *Journal of Clinical Psychiatry*, **66**:7 (2005), 870–86.

43. Sachs G S, Printz D J, Kahn D A, Carpenter D & Docherty J P. The Expert Consensus Guideline Series: medication treatment of bipolar disorder 2000. *Postgraduate Medicine*, Apr 2000; Spec No:1–104.

44. Goodwin G M, Consensus Group of the British Association for Psychopharmacology. Evidence-based guidelines for treating bipolar disorder: revised second edition – recommendations from the British Association for Psychopharmacology. *Journal of Psychopharmacology*, **23**:4 (2009), 346–88.

45. Anon. APA Practice guideline for the treatment of patients with bipolar disorder (revision). *American Journal of Psychiatry*, **159**:4 Suppl (2002), 1–50.

46. Fountoulakis K, Vieta E, Sanchez-Moreno J *et al.* Treatment guidelines for bipolar disorder: a critical review. *Journal of Affective Disorders*, **86**:1 (2005), 1–10.

47. American Psychiatric Association. Practice guideline for the treatment of patients with bipolar disorder, second edition. *American Journal of Psychiatry*, **159**:4 Suppl (2002), 1–50.

48. Hirschfeld R. *Guideline Watch: Practice Guideline for the Treatment of Patients with Bipolar Disorder*. Arlington, VA: American Psychiatric Association; 2005.

49. Carney S & Goodwin G. Lithium – a continuing story in the treatment of bipolar disorder. *Acta Psychiatrica Scandinavica*, **111**:s426 (2005), 7–12.

50. Masters K. Anti-suicidal and self-harm properties of lithium carbonate. *CNS Spectrums*, **13**:2 (2008), 109.

51. Casher M & Bostwick J. Lithium: using the comeback drug. *Current Psychiatry*, 7:5 (2008), 59–60.

52. Rowe M & Chuang D. Lithium neuroprotection: molecular mechanisms and clinical implications. *Expert Reviews in Molecular Medicine*, **6**:21 (2004), 1–18.

53. Carroll B, Thalassinos A & Fawver J. Loading strategies in acute mania. *CNS Spectrums*, **6**:11 (2001), 919–30.

54. Fava G, Molnar G, Block B, Lee J & Perini G. The lithium loading dose method in a clinical setting. *American Journal of Psychiatry*, **141**:6 (1984), 812.

55. Calabrese J, Shelton M, Rapport D *et al*. A 20-month, double-blind, maintenance trial of lithium versus divalproex in rapid-cycling bipolar disorder. *American Journal of Psychiatry*, **162**:11 (2005), 2152.

56. Miller B, Perry W, Moutier C, Robinson S & Feifel D. Rapid oral loading of extended release divalproex in patients with acute mania. *General Hospital Psychiatry*, **27**:3 (2005), 218–21.

57. DRUGDEX®System. www.thomsonhc.com [Accessed October 3, 2009].

58. May T & Rambeck B. Serum concentrations of valproic acid: influence of dose and comedication. *Therapeutic Drug Monitoring*, **7** (1985), 387–90.

59. Cramer J, Mattson R, Bennett D & Swick C. Variable free and total valproic acid concentrations in sole-and multi-drug therapy. *Therapeutic Drug Monitoring*, **8**:4 (1986), 411.

60. Dasgupta A. Clinical utility of free drug monitoring. *Clinical Chemistry and Laboratory Medicine*, **40**:10 (2002), 986–93.

61. Vasudev K, Goswami U & Kohli K. Carbamazepine and valproate monotherapy: feasibility, relative safety and efficacy, and therapeutic drug monitoring in manic disorder. *Psychopharmacology*, **150**:1 (2000), 15–23.

62. Calabrese J, Kimmel S, Woyshville M *et al*. Clozapine for treatment-refractory mania. *American Journal of Psychiatry*, **153**:6 (1996), 759.

63. Mukherjee S, Sackeim H & Schnur D. Electroconvulsive therapy of acute manic episodes: a review of 50 years' experience. *American Journal of Psychiatry*, **151**:2 (1994), 169.

64. Detweiler M B, Mehra A, Rowell T *et al*. Delirious mania and malignant catatonia: a report of 3 cases and review. *Psychiatric Quarterly*, **80**:1 (2009), 23–40.

65. McInnis M. Personal Communication. Ann Arbor, MI; 2009.

66. Saunders E, Langenecker S & McInnis M. Mood-independent and mood-potentiated personality traits in the Prechter bipolar sample. (*under review*). 2008.

67. Üçok A, Karaveli D, Kundakçi T & Yazici O. Comorbidity of personality disorders with bipolar mood disorders. *Comprehensive Psychiatry*, **39**:2 (1998), 72–4.

68. Brieger P, Ehrt U & Marneros A. Frequency of co-morbid personality disorders in bipolar and unipolar affective disorders. *Comprehensive Psychiatry*, **44**:1 (2003), 28–34.

69. Andreasen N. Creativity and mental illness: prevalence rates in writers and their first-degree relatives. *American Journal of Psychiatry*, **144**:10 (1987), 1288.

70. Simeonova D, Chang K, Strong C & Ketter T. Creativity in familial bipolar disorder. *Journal of Psychiatric Research*, **39**:6 (2005), 623–31.

71. Rothenberg A. Bipolar illness, creativity, and treatment. *Psychiatric Quarterly*, **72**:2 (2001), 131–47.

72. Yatham L, Kennedy S, O'Donovan C *et al.* Canadian Network for Mood and Anxiety Treatments (CANMAT) guidelines for the management of patients with bipolar disorder: consensus and controversies. *Bipolar Disorders Supplement*, **7** (2005), 5.

73. Pollack L. Inpatient self-management of bipolar disorder. *Applied Nursing Research*, **9**:2 (1996), 71–9.

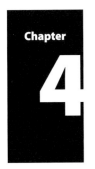

The inpatient with borderline personality disorder

When specific diagnoses are mentioned, we are referring to diagnoses and criteria as listed in the *Diagnostic and Statistical Manual of Mental Disorders*, 4th edition, text revision (DSM-IV-TR) unless otherwise specified.

Why does this particular personality disorder get so much attention?

Patients who fall under the diagnostic heading of borderline personality disorder (BPD) consume a disproportionate percentage of mental health services, are frequent visitors to psychiatric emergency departments (12% of all visits) and to psychiatric units (present in 15 to 18% of inpatients) [1]. Examples and characteristics of this disorder are often included in psychiatric writings on "the difficult patient." (Perhaps *the* classic example of this is the Groves' paper "Taking care of the hateful patient" [2]). They stir up extremes of feeling in caregivers because of their dangerous behaviors, unstable emotions, and intense likes and dislikes – as illustrated by what one psychiatrist said about his work with borderline patients:

> When a patient with BPD is admitted to me in the hospital, I draw a deep breath and tell myself that this is going to be a difficult patient. I prepare myself to go through phases of thinking of myself as a great psychiatrist, alternating with feeling frustrated and hating the patient. I know I will have to spend a lot of time with staff. Some of them will want to get the patient out right away and may get upset with me if this doesn't happen. [3]

This sort of honest appraisal of the challenges of working with patients with BPD is common in experienced clinicians. Indeed, the clinician caring for a patient with BPD will need to talk with others about the case, and will be spending extra time processing various points of view and disparate feelings of the unit staff [4, 5]. In this regard, BPD patients are generally very "labor intensive." They require providers to draw upon all of their clinical skills.

What is the current understanding of the neurobiology and etiology of BPD?

Borderline personality disorder can be viewed as a heterogeneous illness with interplay between constitutional predisposition, i.e., temperament, and environmental factors. Genetics is known to play a role in the trait of emotional dysregulation, and BPD itself is inheritable as suggested by the concordance rate of 35% in monozygotic twins versus 7% in dizygotic twins [6]. Brain abnormalities have been demonstrated in BPD. Neuroimaging findings clearly differentiate BPD subjects from controls, especially in relation to decreased hippocampal, amygdalar, left orbitofrontal, and right anterior cingulate cortical volumes in BPD patients [7, 8]. Functional imaging studies have shown hyperactivation of the amygdala in response to emotional stimuli [9], a neurobiological pattern that is likely associated with the BPD core symptom of emotional dysregulation.

The environmental causal factors include childhood neglect, abuse (physical or sexual), and/or a mismatch between the child's vulnerability and the parents' abilities to maintain a positive attachment in spite of their child's emotional reactivity. Adverse triggering events in later childhood and adolescence also figure in the final pathway toward adult BPD [10].

Psychiatric writings relevant to the etiology and phenomenology of BPD are too abundant to review here in any comprehensive fashion, but a few figures that have enriched the understanding of BPD should be mentioned. From the British Psychoanalytical Society, the contributions of D. W. Winnicott [11–13] and Michael Balint [14] add to current conceptualizations of BPD. These two psychoanalysts treated patients with "primitive character structures" – "borderline features" in current parlance. Winnicott's concept of "good-enough mothering," which describes the parent's creation of a "holding environment" that balances the child's needs for nurturance and independence, has echoes in the way experienced therapists today approach their patients with BPD [12]. The psychiatric inpatient unit, where patients' emotions are allowed expression in a safe and structured fashion, also can be viewed as a kind of "holding environment." Winnicott also coined the term "transitional object" to refer to the blankets and stuffed animals that children use for comfort during the developmental process of separation from the mother [13]. It is interesting to note that some psychiatrists view the presence of a teddy bear on the bed of an adult inpatient as virtually pathognomonic of BPD [15]. Balint presaged modern BPD concepts with his writings about a "basic fault" that develops when insufficient maternal attention to the child's needs results in a sense of emptiness and defect. While his delineation has reverberations in current thinking about BPD, current views of BPD would include the contribution of neurobiological factors in forming this "defect."

More recently, Otto Kernberg, Gerald Adler and Daniel Buie, and John Gunderson made seminal contributions to the psychodynamic understanding of BPD. Kernberg is especially known for the concept of "splitting," which refers to the tendency of patients with BPD to see the world, including the self and others, in black and white terms [16]. This cognitive style represents a failure to integrate experiences of frustration and satisfaction so that the self and others can be viewed in a more nuanced and balanced way. On the inpatient unit, "splitting" may take the form of a patient with BPD getting along extremely well with the day nurses but butting heads with the nighttime staff. Adler and Buie emphasize deficits in early mothering that are reflected in the BPD patient's defect in "object constancy," the ability to evoke a mental image of a comforting person when under stress [17]. This defect in self-soothing is often implicated in the hospital admission of suicidal BPD patients when their outpatient therapists are on vacation. Gunderson sees attachment disturbance as primary in BPD and views the pathology as arising from the mother's emotional abandonment of the child during the separation–individuation process [18, 19]. In addition, Gunderson has been a leading spokesperson for recognition of BPD and the need for increased research into the disorder. In reviewing our current knowledge of BPD and the evolution of the concept over the past seven decades, he concluded that BPD belongs on Axis I rather than Axis II in the upcoming DSM-V [20].

Because of the high co-morbidity of BPD with affective symptoms, some psychiatrists view the symptoms of BPD as a form of bipolar disorder, or as a biological defect in affect regulation [21]. In partial support of this argument, it is striking to note that many of the medications that are useful in BPD are also effective in treatment for affective disorders [22, 23]. However, there are many aspects of BPD that are not accounted for when one views it as a form of bipolar disorder. In addition, adherence to a pure biological view of BPD tends to be associated with an over-reliance on psychopharmacologic approaches that are only partially effective (see below). Another critique of the BPD diagnosis involves the argument that childhood abuse is responsible for BPD, and therefore BPD is actually a sub-set of post-traumatic stress disorder (PTSD), a diagnosis that is also less stigmatizing [24]. However, although childhood sexual abuse is frequently associated with BPD, a history of abuse is not found in all patients with BPD [25]. Furthermore, most BPD patients do not experience the flashbacks, nightmares, and intrusive memories that characterize PTSD.

Under what circumstances would a BPD patient require an admission to an inpatient unit?

A patient with BPD is not likely to be admitted to the unit electively; rather, hospital admission tends to occur when the patient is acutely suicidal or acting out in dangerous ways. Many of these patients suffer with chronic suicidality, making it difficult to determine when the situation has reached a critical point that warrants hospitalization. There have even been arguments advanced that the hospitalization of the patient with BPD does more harm than good, fostering dependency and regression in the patient without putting any serious dent in their longitudinal risk of suicide [26]. Nonetheless, mental health clinicians on the front lines, such as emergency departments and medical-surgical units, still have to contend with patients in escalating cycles of self-harm, and who, in the view of the authors, can benefit from a brief stay on an inpatient unit. For instance, an admission may be necessary if a patient who is usually a "light cutter" has cut more deeply, perhaps injuring an artery or tendon. Another, otherwise stable, patient may have a serious overdose in response to a break-up. Perhaps a patient is increasingly involved in self-destructive sexual behaviors that are not necessarily part of his/her usual pattern. All of these escalating behaviors could be evidence that something new has been injected into the mix. A brief admission allows for de-escalation, necessary medical follow-up, a "booster" of coping skills work with staff, and examination of external factors that might be modifiable to help the patient return to the outpatient treatment setting in good condition.

Patients with BPD have been described as being "stably unstable." In other words, due to problems in adapting to stress, they are generally at risk for a decline in functioning and a significant change in behavior when they encounter situations that they cannot integrate or process. Search for the cause of the current hospitalization will lead to the important "why now?" question in the initial evaluation, but the clinician will have to keep in mind that the patient may not have conscious awareness of the answer. Suffice it to say that the patient's equilibrium has now been shifted by something. It could be something as simple as a change in a medication, or something as hidden as an anticipated threat of abandonment by an idealized figure. Hospitalization becomes an external structure that is needed temporarily to shore up a patient's weak coping apparatus and to augment the patient's deficient "self-soothing" capacity.

What are the elements of the diagnostic interview when a diagnosis of BPD is suspected?

Much useful diagnostic information can be gained with a less structured interview and open-ended questions, at least at first. This allows the clinician to see how the patient structures the interaction. The interpersonal relationship that develops between the patient and the provider has its own diagnostic validity. Some experts in the field put great stock in the interviewer's countertransference reaction, since these patients can rapidly evoke very powerful feelings in the interviewer. One experienced clinician has noted, "If you sit with the patient for five minutes and want to marry them or murder them, the patient is borderline!" [27].

Table 4.1 DSM-IV-TR criteria for Borderline Personality Disorder (abbreviated)

Efforts to avoid real or imagined abandonment

Unstable and intense interpersonal relationships

Identity disturbance, unstable self-image or sense of self

Impulsivity in at least two areas that are potentially self-damaging (not including next line)

Recurrent suicidal behavior, gestures, or threats; or self-mutilating behavior

Affective instability, marked reactivity of mood

Chronic feelings of emptiness

Inappropriate, intense anger or difficulty controlling anger

Transient, stress-related paranoid ideation or severe dissociative symptoms

During the interview, it is useful to keep in mind the major categories of dysfunction that are seen with BPD. Most clinicians utilize the DSM-IV-TR criteria in forming a diagnosis of BPD (Table 4.1). Accordingly, they may have to formulate structured questions that tap into areas that were not covered in the unstructured portion of the interview.

During the interview the clinician should inquire into the patient's ability to manage anger, the patient's sensitivity to abandonment, and the quality of the patient's relationships, both currently and historically. Are the patient's relationships based on mutuality or are the persons deemed "friends" really just "need-satisfying figures?" It is also important to get an overall idea of how the patient has functioned over the course of his or her life. The clinician should try to come away from the interview with a portrayal of how the patient has interacted with the world, and how the patient has managed the inevitable stresses of life. A BPD diagnosis should be considered if the patient presents a picture of waxing and waning periods of unhappiness and psychiatric symptoms occurring over a period of years, a high level of emotional reactivity and impulsivity, and the lack of a clear path in life with regard to schooling, career, and relationships. A useful mnemonic to recall the categories of chronic dysfunction in BPD is shown in Table 4.2.

When evaluating a patient with possible BPD, ancillary information from family members or a significant other, past records, and current caregivers is always helpful. Patients may resist the inpatient team's request to speak with family members. They may be trying to avoid exposing disparities between their own and the family's accounts of the history. This can occur in particular when the patient's symptoms are ego-syntonic. In addition, treating BPD inpatients in a vacuum with no contact with family prevents the clinician from learning about the people to which the patient is returning following the

Table 4.2 IMPULSIVE – a mnemonic for BPD [28]

I	Impulsive
M	Moodiness
P	Paranoia (or dissociation) under stress
U	Unstable self-image
L	Labile, intense relationships
S	Suicidal gestures
I	Inappropriate anger
V	Vulnerability to abandonment
E	Emptiness (feelings of…)

hospitalization. It is useful to know how the family views the patient, and how much support the patient will have after discharge. Similar considerations apply if the patient is receiving significant support from persons outside the family, including staff at a group home, or friends who spend a lot of time with the patient. Their input can be extremely valuable for treatment and disposition planning.

How important is it to examine for co-morbid conditions in patients with BPD?

Though personality disorders in DSM are supposedly enduring across the adult lifespan, in clinical practice we find that the symptoms and signs of BPD may fluctuate in severity over time – even remit to the point where a patient is no longer "borderline" – depending upon a variety of internal and external circumstances [29, 30]. Co-morbid disorders and recent stressors can push the patient toward the lower level of their range of functioning and can destabilize the patient with BPD who had gained some equilibrium through therapy, medications, or from maturation. For many patients then, it is not sufficient to make the diagnosis of BPD alone; a search for co-morbid illness should be an important part of the evaluation.

Patients with BPD have a high probability of having a number of Axis I disorders that interfere with gaining stability in outpatient treatment [30, 31]. Identifying and beginning treatment for co-occurring disorders on the inpatient unit is important. Common co-morbid conditions are bipolar disorder, major depressive disorder, dysthymia, PTSD, eating disorders, pathological gambling, dissociative disorders, ADHD, and somatoform disorders (Figure 4.1). An Axis I mood disorder diagnosis can be particularly hard to make if clouded by the affective instability and feelings of emptiness that are

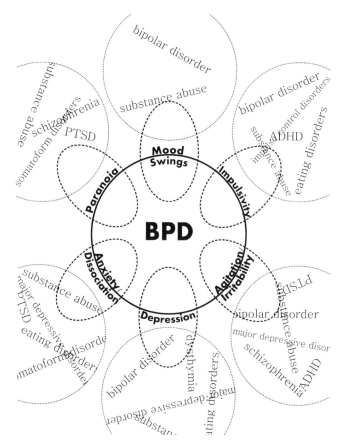

Figure 4.1 Overlap of borderline personality disorder (BPD) symptom-clusters with Axis I disorders.

part of BPD itself. It is useful here to distinguish relatively brief, stressor-driven affective dysregulation from the more enduring, autonomously driven moods of a primary mood disorder. While it is true that self-mutilation is very often a symptom of BPD, if a 40-year-old patient who has been in treatment for BPD for 20 years gets depressed and starts cutting, a new onset primary mood disorder should be suspected.

Finally, medical illness can knock a stable BPD patient off balance, so an initial physical examination and routine blood work, including thyroid testing, are necessary. Furthermore, since all patients with BPD are at risk for using substances, a blood alcohol level and urine drug screen should be part of the initial evaluation. Addictions can undermine even the most well conceived outpatient therapy set up. If a patient with BPD is using drugs or alcohol, the symptoms of impulsivity and affect dysregulation may increase.

What is the relationship between psychosis and BPD?

Transient paranoid reactions related to stress can occur in BPD and are included in DSM criteria for the disorder. Past writers have referred to these as "micro-" or "quasi-psychotic episodes" [32, 33]. Auditory hallucinations are not part of the typical BPD picture, and when reported, generally have a different quality to those seen in schizophrenia. They may actually represent over-valued thoughts experienced by the patient as "voices." In other instances they may even be a factitious "ticket for admission" to the hospital [34]. If a full-blown, non-transient psychosis is seen in a patient with BPD, a co-occurring psychotic disorder or substance use should be strongly considered.

How does the inpatient approach to BPD differ from the outpatient approach?

At the present time, the majority of the treatment of a patient with BPD takes place in an outpatient setting, and may include dialectical behavioral therapy (DBT) (see below). The outpatient treatment might be punctuated with brief, hopefully infrequent, periods of time spent on general psychiatric inpatient units during times of crisis. When the care of the patient with BPD is structured in this fashion, it is important that any inpatient stay be brief and focused, and not overly ambitious in its goals [35]. Inpatient clinicians get into trouble when they take on the patient's whole borderline personality structure, or set as a goal the elimination of an entrenched behavior, such as self-cutting. Rather, the hospital goals should be structured around patient safety, with therapeutic interactions and medication management centered on increasing the patient's ability to cope with whatever stressors led to the admission. If the patient cannot set a specific short-term goal for the brief hospitalization, the goal becomes – by default – "learning how to set a short-term goal." The hospital can be a place where the clinician begins a dialogue with the patient about alternatives to the ways he or she is thinking about his or her life. In a related vein, the caregiver can introduce the idea that there may be other ways to cope with the pain the patient is experiencing. This could begin or further a process that will be continued in much greater depth in the outpatient setting. More specifically, many inpatient units are now implementing DBT-based approaches for treatment of BPD patients. These interventions can be individual or be programmed into the group therapy offerings. They range in intensity from a weekly "coping group" to

Table 4.3 *In our experience...* Tips for dealing with the patient with BPD in the hospital

Do not try to fix all the patient's problems during a brief stay. Work on the most pressing current issues.

Set a discharge date early in the admission and try to adhere to it, give or take a day or two.

Avoid the search for the "perfect" medication regimen. Remind the patient (and yourself) that medications are only a small part of the treatment.

Try to stay compassionate, interested, and validating. In DBT terms, this is called "wise mind."

Be willing to negotiate, within limits, on medications, privileges, etc.

Decompress with your treatment team and your colleagues.

If the BPD diagnosis is new to a patient with a co-morbid mood disorder, consider having a "borderline talk" to explain why he/she has been doing so poorly with previous treatments.

Reframe the illness as an "emotional regulation" problem if the patient seems stigmatized by the BPD label.

Remember: You CAN stay calm and centered with BPD patients by focusing your treatment goals and enlisting all team members as active partners

months-long intensive inpatient programs designed to kick-start outpatient DBT [36, 37]. All staff members should have at least basic knowledge of the tenets of DBT. (See Table 4.3.)

When encountering a patient with BPD on the inpatient unit, it may be useful to recall the various ways that BPD has been conceptualized. This may enable the clinician to maintain empathy during the various stormy periods that will arise in the patient's stay on the unit. Many of the interpersonal behaviors that are disruptive to the unit and that make the staff angry are maladaptive survival strategies that the BPD patient has evolved to deal with affective dysregulation and intense feelings of pain. Being cognizant of BPD patients' propensity towards splitting, their difficulties in self-soothing, their problems in recognizing their own feelings, and their need to feel "validated," will shape the way one interacts with BPD patients on the unit.

Can BPD be treated with psychotherapy?

Responding to the need for a treatment that addresses repeated suicidal behaviors, Marsha Linehan developed DBT, a form of cognitive therapy that is particularly effective in BPD patients [38]. Linehan views borderline pathology as resulting when a child with a constitutional predisposition to react excessively to stress is reared in an "invalidating environment" in which his or her experiences, emotional responses, and communications are not recognized, affirmed, and supported by parenting figures. A one-year prospective study comparing DBT with "treatment as usual" found that the DBT group had fewer days of inpatient hospitalization, a decreased number of suicide attempts, and were more likely to remain in treatment [39].

In recent years, Anthony Bateman and Peter Fonagy have developed a manualized psychotherapy based on "mentalization" [40]. Mentalization is the ability to recognize one's own mental states and those of others. The theoretical basis for the treatment is that patients with BPD are deficient in this ability. The capacity to mentalize is a developmental accomplishment that requires a stable attachment to primary parenting figures in early childhood. Disruptions and impediments in this pathway are thought to contribute to adult psychopathology [41]. The work of Bateman and Fonagy meshes easily with other therapeutic approaches that emphasize the formation of a secure attachment to a therapist who "corrects" the maladaptive beliefs and cognitions that have arisen from deficits in development.

How might psychotherapeutic approaches be applied during a brief inpatient stay?

All the elements of good inpatient treatment – meaningful team meetings, unified approach to the patient, attention to boundary issues, and a structured program of groups and activities – are especially important with BPD patients. Because of their own fragmented self-concept, patients with BPD do best when expectations are carefully outlined, and do less well when there are "fracture lines" in the treatment milieu. The clinician should strive to have good communication with all the members of the team and should be prepared for differences in opinion about the patient's presentation, when to advance privileges, and how much conscious control the patient has over his or her actions.

If psychiatric unit staff gain familiarity with the fundamentals of DBT, mentalization, or both, episodes of acting out by a patient on the unit can be managed by using these principles and skills. Although a short-term hospital model may not allow more than an introduction to some of these ideas, groups on the unit can begin this process. Dialectical behavioral therapy, for example, has four sets of skills: mindfulness, interpersonal effectiveness, emotional modulation, and distress tolerance [38]. Very basic overviews of these skills and their application to crisis management can be provided to psychiatric inpatients via group sessions even where the typical length of stay is a week or less. Furthermore, these concepts are useful for any person in crisis or trying to handle difficult emotions, so staff should be encouraged to make the material widely available. Even more practically, a given incident on the unit, e.g., a patient curses angrily at a nurse, can be subjected to a "chain analysis," which will outline the sequence of feelings and events that led to the outburst. This in turn can lead to reflection with the patient about the DBT skills that could have been used to prevent a situation from escalating.

What is the role of medication in the treatment of patients with BPD?

Most patients with BPD have had multiple "off-label" trials of various medications in attempts to mute the behavioral dyscontrol, the affective lability, and the cognitive distortions that are part of the symptom complex of BPD. At this time there are no medications that are FDA-approved for the treatment of BPD. In fact, the most recent recommendation from the National Institute for Health and Clinical Excellence to the UK's National Health Service is to avoid medication treatments in BPD unless there is a co-morbid psychiatric condition [42]. Sometimes it is hard to resist the entreaties of the patient with BPD for more and more medications, and poorly conceived polypharmacy can result. Nonetheless, the recent work on neurobiological correlates of BPD, and related work on identifying seemingly hard-wired deficits in dimensions such as management of impulsivity and aggression, has lent credence to pharmacologic strategies that target the various domains of impaired functioning in BPD [43]. In addition, hospitalized BPD patients, who have a high likelihood of co-morbid Axis I conditions, will generally benefit from targeted pharmacotherapy. Since many hospitalized patients with BPD will already be on one or more medications, the task of the inpatient psychiatrist may be one of "tweaking" the existing regimen for greater efficacy, reduction of side effects, or both. Patients who are astute about their illness will often describe the effect of medications as a "safety net" that can lessen symptoms and protect against decompensation under stress. The following sections review the classes of medications that have been used in treating BPD and which may help stabilize patients who are admitted to the hospital (Table 4.4) [22, 23].

Antidepressants

Because of the frequent co-morbidity of affective disorders and BPD, it makes sense to use medications that will treat the co-morbid condition simultaneously with the core BPD symptoms. A good example of this would be the use of a selective serotonin reuptake inhibitor (SSRI), which can address primary depressive symptoms while also targeting BPD core symptoms of anger, impulsivity, and irritability. Since this constellation of symptoms is so common, SSRIs are often seen as a first-line agent for BPD. Tricyclic antidepressants (TCAs) are less useful in this regard, and should be avoided due to their lethality in overdose; BPD patients may also be especially sensitive to cognitive impairment due to the anticholinergic effects of TCAs. Monoamine oxidase inhibitors (MAOIs) are often avoided due to fears that the patient with BPD will act out around the dietary restrictions and be at risk for a tyramine

Table 4.4 Medications used for borderline personality disorder symptoms [22, 23, 43–45]

Medication	Comments
SSRIs and SNRIs	useful for depression, anxiety, impulsivity, self-harm
	relatively safe in overdose
	avoid in patients with co-morbid bipolar I or II
Mood stabilizers (lithium, carbamazepine, valproate, lamotrigine, topiramate)	for lability, anger/agitation/aggression, impulsivity
	lithium is the *least* safe of these in overdose
Antipsychotics (typical and atypical)	consider for paranoia/disorganized thinking, dissociation, hostility
	also maybe for lability, anger/agitation/aggression, impulsivity
Benzodiazepines	best to avoid in BPD due to dependency and disinhibition
	still used for acute agitation on many inpatient units
Tricyclic antidepressants	avoid due to lethality in overdose, no evidence for BPD symptoms
	may have to consider in BPD with treatment-resistant depression
MAOIs	many side effects, not first-line
	may consider with atypical symptoms
	early literature on "hysteroid dysphoria" supports use
Naltrexone	may reduce dissociation and self-cutting behavior

reaction. However, for the more reliable patient with BPD, this group of medications may be helpful with the atypical depression and rejection sensitivity that are commonly observed with BPD. Bupropion may have a role for a BPD patient with co-morbid attention-deficit/hyperactivity disorder (ADHD) and substance use, a situation in which the use of abusable stimulants would not be desirable.

Table 4.5 Typical doses of some antipsychotic medications used in borderline personality disorder

Risperidone	0.5 to 1.0 mg per day
Quetiapine	25 to 100 mg per day
Olanzapine	2.5 to 5.0 mg per day
Aripiprazole	2.5 to 10 mg per day
Ziprasidone	20 to 40 mg per day, up to 80 mg twice a day
Trifluoperazine	2 to 8 mg per day
Thiothixine	2 to 4 mg per day, in divided doses

Antipsychotics

Both typical and atypical antipsychotics have been used in BPD, with the latter group now supplanting the former. Low doses are generally the rule with either, as shown in Table 4.5 [43]. This class of medication is considered for the BPD symptoms in the "cognitive–perceptual" domain, including transient psychotic or psychotic-like states, and paranoia. They also may be useful for dissociative symptoms, which are often driven by intense "pan-anxiety." In addition, antipsychotics can mute the symptoms of hostility and aggression in BPD. When patients balk at the idea of taking a "schizophrenia medicine," they may need to hear that the medication is being used "off- label" as a "major tranquilizer."

Mood stabililizers/anticonvulsants

This group of medications can be used to target the affective dysregulation and impulsive behavioral dyscontrol clusters of symptoms [46]. One can generally make a distinction between the affective swings in BPD, which tend to be more reactive to events, and the more autonomous mood swings of bipolar disorder. Nonetheless, there is considerable overlap in the medications used to treat both kinds of mood instability. In addition, these medications will be particularly helpful for BPD patients with co-occurring bipolar disorder.

Lithium can be helpful with BPD mood instability, and has anti-suicidal properties that add to the benefits for BPD. However, lithium use requires a solid therapeutic relationship because of this medication's narrow therapeutic index and the potential for lethal overdose. Carbamazepine and valproate have both been used with some benefit for impulsivity and behavioral dyscontrol. More recently, lamotrigine and topiramate (two medications that are also weight neutral) have shown usefulness for anger and aggression in BPD. Gabapentin can serve as an alternative to benzodiazepines (which should be avoided if possible in BPD) for anxiety-related symptoms [22].

Opioid antagonists

Some clinicians who work with patients with BPD, and some open-ended studies, have found that naltrexone can decrease the frequency of cutting behavior and the associated craving to cut. The theoretical basis underlying this effect of opioid antagonists is the idea that BPD patients have abnormalities in their opiate system leading to impaired pain processing. These medications may be more effective when there is an element of dissociation and lack of pain awareness with the cutting [45]. Naltrexone should be seen as an adjunct to therapies such as DBT that are directed at developing coping strategies to deal with suicidality, and which have a more proven track record for prevention of suicidal and parasuicidal behaviors.

What is the best way to deal with BPD patients' suicidality on an inpatient unit?

Patients with BPD have a high incidence of "parasuicidal" behaviors that are generally not fatal, such as self-cutting, self-burning, and overdosing on non-lethal amounts of medications. However, over their lifespan patients with BPD do have a 3 to 10% risk of completed suicide [1]. At some point – during a hospitalization may be the best time – the patient's loved ones should be told about the long-term mortality risk associated with this illness. This frank, unpleasant discussion can be coupled with a review of more optimistic data on the favorable long-term prognosis of BPD patients who engage in, and remain in, appropriate treatment [39].

Because suicidal feelings or actions often are the reason for admission to an inpatient unit, the patient needs to be continually assessed for suicide risk during clinical interviews. Many patients with BPD are chronically suicidal and will say that they cannot give up the suicidal ideas, which represent a kind of "trick up their sleeve," or serve a soothing function at times of stress. Repetitive self-cutting has a similar purpose for many patients. Suicidal threats and actions in BPD can also be highly interpersonal in nature, and may be attempts to engage significant others and to "extract" care from family and friends – and clinicians. Generally, though, when a BPD patient requires admission to the hospital, there has been a change in the nature of the suicidality, perhaps even to the point where a patient who previously only had general thoughts about committing suicide reports that he or she now has a specific plan. The hospital can be the temporary "holding environment," discussed above, where the patient can figure out what factors have altered a pre-existing homeostasis. When suicidal and parasuicidal acting out continues on the inpatient unit, the need for close monitoring to assure safety will need to be balanced against the risk of prolonging the inpatient stay and of undermining the patient's responsibility for self-control. Targeted pharmacotherapy may be useful in these instances, but more crucial will be therapies on the inpatient unit that direct the patient toward ways of coping with the increased hopeless feelings rather than acting upon them.

How is the co-ordination of inpatient treatment with the outpatient team handled?

When a patient with BPD is on an inpatient psychiatric unit, the inpatient clinicians have a consultative role vis-à-vis the current outpatient treatment clinician or team. While the patient may have "requested" the consultation, i.e., by coming to the emergency department, *without* the prior knowledge of the outpatient treatment provider(s), the inpatient team should not make major revisions to the treatment plan without communicating with the patient's primary therapist. It is true that the hospitalization offers a chance for a "fresh look" at the patient and the efficacy of the current outpatient treatment approach, but a few misplaced words from an inpatient clinician can undermine months or even years of work between the patient and the outpatient provider.

That said, it is indeed important to tactfully determine the quality of the therapeutic alliance with the outpatient psychiatrist or therapist, not only from the patient's point of view but from that of the outpatient provider as well. If that therapist appears to have a reasonable relationship with the patient, and if he or she is feeling overwhelmed and frustrated with the patient's behaviors, the inpatient clinician or team can offer reassurance. Admission of the BPD patient to the hospital can even seem like a kind of respite for the outpatient clinician, since he or she not only gets to share some likely negative thoughts or feelings with a colleague, but, at least for a brief time, the patient is "safe" and not his or her direct responsibility.

On the other hand, if the outpatient therapist does not have a good alliance with the patient, or the therapy seems to be unhelpful or harmful, then the inpatient consultant must decide how much to interfere. For example, if the outpatient caregiver is not aware of the available treatments, such as DBT, the inpatient clinician might mention, "I've really gotten into DBT for this kind of patient. It can really help with regressions." This is very treacherous territory, especially given the intensity of affect involved with BPD and the amount of chaos already in these patients' lives. Despite the best efforts of the inpatient team, the patient may end up returning to sub-optimal or sub-standard treatment. This should be documented in the record and may serve as a "red flag" should a readmission be considered during a future emergency department visit.

Finally, some outpatient therapists or psychiatrists may use the patient's hospitalization as an opportunity to bow out gracefully from an unworkable situation with a difficult BPD patient. In general this should be respected and efforts made to secure different post-discharge treatment for the patient.

References

1. Gunderson J & Links P. *Borderline Personality Disorder: A Clinical Guide.* American Psychiatric Pub; 2008.

2. Groves J E. Taking care of the hateful patient. *New England Journal of Medicine*, **298**:16 (1978), 883–7.

3. Gimbel B. Personal communication. Ann Arbor, MI; 2008.

4. Deans C & Meocevic E. Attitudes of registered psychiatric nurses towards patients diagnosed with borderline personality disorder. *Contemporary Nurse*, **21**:1 (2006), 43–9.

5. Rossberg J, Karterud S, Pedersen G & Friis S. An empirical study of countertransference reactions toward patients with personality disorders. *Comprehensive Psychiatry*, **48**:3 (2007), 225–30.

6. Lieb K, Zanarini M, Schmahl C, Linehan M & Bohus M. Borderline personality disorder. *The Lancet*, **364**:9432 (2004), 453–61.

7. Brambilla P, Soloff P H, Sala M *et al.* Anatomical MRI study of borderline personality disorder patients. *Psychiatry Research*, **131**:2 (2004), 125–33.

8. Tebartz van Elst L, Hesslinger B, Thiel T *et al.* Frontolimbic brain abnormalities in patients with borderline personality disorder: a volumetric magnetic resonance imaging study. *Biological Psychiatry*, **54**:2 (2003), 163–71.

9. Donegan N H, Sanislow C A, Blumberg H P *et al.* Amygdala hyperreactivity in borderline personality disorder: implications for emotional dysregulation. *Biological Psychiatry*, **54**:11 (2003), 1284–93.

10. Zanarini M C & Frankenburg F R. Pathways to the development of borderline personality disorder. *Journal of Personality Disorders*, **11**:1 (1997), 93–104.

11. Sadock B J, Sadock V A, Kaplan H I. *Kaplan & Sadock's Comprehensive Textbook of Psychiatry*, 8th edn. Philadelphia, PA: Lippincott Williams & Wilkins; 2004.

12. Winnicott D. The capacity to be alone. *International Journal of Psycho-Analysis*, **39** (1958), 416–20.

13. Winnicott D W. Transitional objects and transitional phenomena; a study of the first not-me possession. *International Journal of Psycho-Analysis*, **34**:2 (1953), 89–97.

14. Balint M & Ornstein P. *The Basic Fault: the Therapeutic Aspects of Regression.* Evanston, IL: Evanston Northwestern University Press; 1968.

15. Cardasis W, Hochman J & Silk K. Transitional objects and borderline personality disorder. *American Journal of Psychiatry*, **154**:2 (1997), 250–5.

16. Kernberg O. *Borderline Conditions and Pathological Narcissism.* New York: Jason Aronson; 1975.

17. Adler G & Buie D H Jr. Aloneness and borderline psychopathology: the possible relevance of child development issues. *International Journal of Psycho-Analysis*, **60**:1 (1979), 83–96.

18. Gunderson J. *Borderline Personality Disorder*. Washington DC: American Psychiatric Press; 1984.

19. Gunderson J G. The borderline patient's intolerance of aloneness: insecure attachments and therapist availability. *American Journal of Psychiatry*, **153**:6 (1996), 752–8.

20. Gunderson J G. Borderline personality disorder: ontogeny of a diagnosis. *American Journal of Psychiatry*, **166**:5 (2009), 530–9.

21. MacKinnon D & Pies R. Affective instability as rapid cycling: theoretical and clinical implications for borderline personality and bipolar spectrum disorders. *Bipolar Disorders*, **8**:1 (2006), 1.

22. Grossman R. Psychopharmacologic treatment of patients with borderline personality disorder. *Psychiatric Annals*, **32**:6 (2002), 357–72.

23. Triebwasser J & Siever L. Pharmacotherapy of personality disorders. *Journal of Mental Health*, **16**:1 (2007), 5–50.

24. Becker D. When she was bad: borderline personality disorder in a posttraumatic age. *American Journal of Orthopsychiatry*, **70** (2000), 4.

25. Bradley R, Jenei J & Westen D. Etiology of borderline personality disorder: disentangling the contributions of intercorrelated antecedents. *Journal of Nervous & Mental Disease*, **193**:1 (2005), 24–31.

26. Paris J. Is hospitalization useful for suicidal patients with borderline personality disorder? *Journal of Personality Disorders*, **18**:3 Special issue (2004), 240–7.

27. Silk K R. Personal communication. Ann Arbor, MI; 2008.

28. Senger H L. Borderline mnemonic. *American Journal of Psychiatry*, **154**:9 (1997), 1321.

29. Sansone R & Sansone L. A longitudinal perspective on personality disorder symptomatology. *Psychiatry*, **5**:1 (2008), 53–61.

30. Zanarini M C, Frankenburg F R, Dubo E D *et al.* Axis I comorbidity of borderline personality disorder. *American Journal of Psychiatry*, **155**:12 (1998), 1733–9.

31. Zanarini M C, Frankenburg F R, Hennen J, Reich D B & Silk K R. Axis I comorbidity in patients with borderline personality disorder: 6-year follow-up and prediction of time to remission. *American Journal of Psychiatry*, **161**:11 (2004), 2108–14.

32. Paris J. Borderline personality disorder. *Canadian Medical Association Journal*, **172**:12 (2005), 1579.

33. Zanarini M, Gunderson J & Frankenburg F. Cognitive features of borderline personality disorder. *American Journal of Psychiatry*, **147**:1 (1990), 57.

34. Pope H Jr, Jonas J & Jones B. Factitious psychosis: phenomenology, family history, and long-term outcome of nine patients. *American Journal of Psychiatry*, **139**:11 (1982), 1480–3.

35. Silk K, Eisner W & Allport C *et al.* Focused time-limited inpatient treatment of borderline personality disorder. *Journal of Personality Disorders*, **8** (1994), 268–78.

36. Bohus M, Haaf B, Stiglmayr C *et al.* Evaluation of inpatient dialectical-behavioral therapy for borderline personality disorder – a prospective study. *Behaviour Research and Therapy*, **38** (2000), 875–87.

37. Swenson C, Sanderson C, Dulit R & Linehan M. The application of dialectical behavior therapy for patients with borderline personality disorder on inpatient units. *Psychiatric Quarterly*, **72**:4 (2001), 307–24.

38. Linehan M. *The Skills Training Manual for Treating Borderline Personality Disorder.* New York: Guilford Press; 1993.

39. Linehan M. The empirical basis of dialectical behavior therapy: development of new treatments versus evaluation of existing treatments. *Clinical Psychology Science and Practice*, **7**:1 (2000), 113–19.

40. Bateman A & Fonagy P. *Psychotherapy for Borderline Personality Disorder: Mentalization-based Treatment.* Oxford: Oxford University Press; 2004.

41. Choi-Kain L W & Gunderson J G. Mentalization: ontogeny, assessment, and application in the treatment of borderline personality disorder. *American Journal of Psychiatry*, **165**:9 (2008), 1127–35.

42. National Institute for Health and Clinical Excellence (NICE). *Borderline Personality Disorder: Treatment and Management (CG 78).* NICE: London; 2009.

43. Saunders E & Silk K. Personality trait dimensions and the pharmacological treatment of borderline personality disorder. *Journal of Clinical Psychopharmacology*, **29**:5 (2009), 461.

44. Kayser A, Robinson D, Nies A & Howard D. Response to phenelzine among depressed patients with features of hysteroid dysphoria. *American Journal of Psychiatry*, **142**:4 (1985), 486.

45. Bohus M, Landwehrmeyer B, Stiglmayr C *et al.* Naltrexone in the treatment of dissociative symptoms in patients with borderline personality disorder: an open-label trial. *Journal of Clinical Psychiatry*, **60**:9 (1999), 598–603.

46. Zanarini M. Antiepileptic drugs and borderline personality disorder. In: McElroy S L, Post R M & Keck P E Jr. eds., *Antiepileptic Drugs to Treat Psychiatric Disorders*. New York: Informa Healthcare, Inc.; 2008, pp. 343–8.

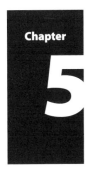

The inpatient with dementia

When specific diagnoses are mentioned, we are referring to diagnoses and criteria as listed in the *Diagnostic and Statistical Manual of Mental Disorders*, 4th edition, text revision (DSM-IV-TR) unless otherwise specified.

Why might a patient with dementia get admitted to the psychiatric inpatient unit?

Dementia is an umbrella term that refers to a group of disorders defined by deterioration in intellectual functioning. Alzheimer's dementia is the proto-typical example, and accounts for some 40 to 60% of all cases of dementia [1]. There are a number of other types of dementia, which present less frequently (Tables 5.1 and 5.2) [2]. A dementia diagnosis requires defects in memory and in at least one other domain of cognitive functioning, such as reasoning ability, visual–spatial processing, mathematical ability, language, or executive func-tion. Aphasia (difficulty with receptive and/or expressive language), apraxia (loss of ability to perform previously learned tasks), and agnosia (misidentifi-cation of familiar people, objects, or places) are also often seen with dementia. In addition to cognitive deficits, dementia is also associated with personality, mood, and behavioral changes. With the incidence of dementia at 5 to 10 % in the general population greater than 65 years old, it is not surprising that a general inpatient psychiatric unit will encounter these patients on a regular basis [1].

Dementia can be associated with a number of acute and sub-acute prob-lems that may lead to psychiatric admission. Some patients are admitted from nursing homes or other extended-care facilities (ECFs) that are no longer able to manage the patient's disruptive behavior. These patients may be frankly psychotic, with delusional thinking and/or hallucinations; confused and/or delirious; or agitated and combative for reasons not related to psychosis or confusion but obviously distressing to the staff and the patient. For instance, a given patient with dementia may start going into other residents' rooms, striking out physically at staff, engaging in inappropriate sexual behavior, or accusing others of stealing items from his or her room. Dementia patients who

Table 5.1 Potentially reversible causes of dementia [2]

Central nervous system infections, e.g., HIV, neurosyphilis, bacterial or fungal meningitis, or viral encephalitis

Normal pressure hydrocephalus

Subdural hematoma

Pernicious anemia

Vasculitis, e.g., that associated with systemic lupus erythematosis

Nutritional deficiencies, e.g., B12 deficiency

Drug toxicity

Pseudodementia, i.e., with depression

Hypothyroidism

require hospitalization may have already had trials of various medications and attempts at behavioral control at the ECF without much success.

Similar situations can occur when a spouse or family members are attempting to care for a dementia patient in the home. The patient may be "sundowning," wandering away from home, or accusing family members of poisoning them – any of which could be leading to caregiver "burn-out" among the involved family members. For these patients, psychiatric hospitalization with a comprehensive evaluation and subsequent stabilization *may* allow the patient's safe return to home. In many instances, though, the hospitalization results in recognition that the needs of the dementia patient outstrip the caregiving capacities of the family, and that placement in a structured facility is needed [3–5].

Depressive syndromes and psychosis are commonly associated with many forms of dementia, and can lead to inability of the patient to care for self, or result in dangerousness to self or others. In most jurisdictions, dementia patients with this level of illness will meet criteria for an involuntary admission to the psychiatric hospital [6]. In some cases, families may have obtained legal guardianship rights that allow them to hospitalize the patient on a psychiatric unit. Some of these dementia patients may have engaged in suicidal actions, and others may have become violent. Still others will represent a hazard to themselves by virtue of not caring for their basic needs, having become so cognitively impaired that they cannot safely manage at home.

Occasionally a patient may be referred to a psychiatric unit by an internist or other primary care physician who has been managing the patient as an outpatient and is now concerned about his/her declining mood or paranoid thought process. In these instances, a psychiatric hospitalization may allow a comprehensive work-up with laboratory testing, imaging and other diagnostic tests, neuropsychological testing, sleep and/or specialist consultation. An inpatient psychiatric unit also provides a monitored environment for trials of psychotropic medication in frail elderly patients who are susceptible to side effects of medications.

Finally, of note, sometimes patients are admitted to the hospital for behavioral problems, psychosis, or mood disorders for which dementia has not yet been considered in the differential diagnosis. In these instances the psychiatric symptoms may be so prominent that the neurocognitive signs of dementia are obscured, and become apparent only in the course of close observation and comprehensive evaluation and treatment on the inpatient unit.

What comprises a comprehensive evaluation of dementia on the inpatient psychiatric unit?

Information gathering is key in formulating a diagnosis and plan. If a patient is arriving from a nursing home, the clinician will need to find out *exactly* what problematic behaviors were occurring at the referring facility. Particular attention should be paid to sleep, appetite, mood, disturbances in thinking, "sundowning," participation in activities, and sociability. It is important to look for precipitating factors and patterns to the behaviors in question.

When interviewing the family, obtaining a detailed time line of the cognitive decline is helpful – though many families may find it difficult to provide one. Functional impairment can occur prior to any decline in performance on the basic cognitive examinations used in primary care offices or general hospitals. Particular attention should be paid to how well the patient is performing basic activities of daily living (ADLs). These include toileting, bathing, feeding, and dressing. Decline in higher level "instrumental" activities of daily living (IADLs) should be a focus of inquiry as well: i.e., the ability to drive or use public transportation, cook one's meals, take medications appropriately, communicate adequately (e.g., name objects and people, use the telephone), and manage one's finances (e.g., balance a checkbook and pay bills). Family can also be asked if they have seen specific depressive symptoms or symptoms of paranoia and psychosis. Finally, people who know the patient well can also assist the clinician in elaborating a more holistic view of the "person" being treated on the inpatient unit by providing information about the patient's hobbies, pre-morbid personality traits, and employment history.

The history also provides a window into some of the more common precipitants that have led a patient with known dementia to regress to the point where hospitalization is needed. Precipitating factors include medication changes, environmental changes (e.g., change in caregiver or room, death of a spouse), occult infection, pain, and sensory deprivation (e.g., worsening visual or hearing impairment, or hemianopsia). A related principle here is that patients with dementia are sensitive to even minor disruptions, can become agitated with alterations in routine, and acclimate slowly to these changes.

As dementia progresses, the collateral sources of information become increasingly important in determining the patient's treatment needs. Useful data are often found in progress notes from the nursing facility, previous medical records, and in historical information from family and caregivers. This information may be the only reliable data to complete all the elements of the standard psychiatric assessment.

An important early task is to establish therapeutic rapport with the patient. This may be difficult in advanced states of dementia, or when the patient is agitated. If the patient has had to sit through a litany of complaints by their family in a combined meeting with family and patient, the patient may be irritable and shut off from talking further. Furthermore, family members, attempting to fill in gaps in the patient's recollections, may repeatedly interrupt the patient's discourse. For these reasons, even patients with moderate degrees of dementia should be interviewed separately, which will serve to validate the patient's portrayal of issues and indirectly communicates the psychiatrist's primary advocacy for the designated patient. Much information is gained by allowing the patient to have some uninterrupted time to relate the story of their illness as they understand it. There is no need to jump in with formal cognitive testing at the onset of the initial interview. Although the overall information from the patient may emerge in a disorganized form, it can be merged with collateral information and put in the proper order in the written evaluation. The interviewer will see that much of what is required to assess the patient's mental status can be accumulated without asking a lot of loaded questions. The initial interview should include bedside cognitive tests. The most frequently used is the Mini-Mental Status Examination (MMSE) [7], although patients with significant cognitive "reserve" may score adequately on this examination in early stages of dementia. More sophistication is added by including additional tests that assess perceptual integration, visual–spatial co-ordination, and frontal circuitry functions and incorporate more executive functioning elements than the MMSE. The Montreal Cognitive Assessment (MoCA) is easy to administer and incorporates a number of executive functioning elements. This test may reveal early dementia and frontal deficits that escape detection with the MMSE [8].

What about a general medical evaluation of the psychiatric inpatient with dementia?

Patients who are in the process of being evaluated for possible dementia will need an extensive work-up to rule out reversible causes of dementia (Table 5.1). Even if the dementia is not in question, a decompensation may be due to an undiagnosed medical problem such as pneumonia or a urinary tract infection. Patients with such medical issues may even present with delirium superimposed on the underlying dementia illness [9]. The review of systems is especially important, with attention to such symptoms as dysuria, cloudy urine, fever, productive cough, and/or recent falls. In cases of moderate or severe cognitive impairment, information from caregivers is essential for a complete investigation of possible medical symptoms. For example, a dementia patient with severe communication impairment will not be able to relay considerable pain from an undiagnosed fracture, which may be suspected only because a family member observes that the patient is favoring or guarding on one side of the body. Medications may also be a culprit in instances of worsening dementia or development of delirium. Opiate pain medications, benzodiazepines, and medications with anticholinergic effects, such as bladder agents and antihistamines, are all "deliriogenic" and can easily destabilize a patient with dementia [10].

A general principle in the inpatient medical evaluation of patients with dementia is to pay particular attention to new physical findings, acute changes in mentation, new behavioral issues, and/or acute personality changes. If the physician makes the mistake of attributing all new findings to known dementia, an underlying general medical disorder can be easily overlooked.

Routine laboratory screening on the inpatient unit of a patient with cognitive or behavioral impairment suspicious for dementia should include complete blood count (CBC), urine analysis (with culture and sensitivity as appropriate), urine drug screen, a comprehensive labaratory panel (including electrolytes, liver functions, calcium, and fasting glucose), B12, folate, thyroid function, magnesium, and syphilis serology [11]. Blood levels of medications the patient is currently taking, such as lithium, phenytoin, or digitalis, should also be obtained. A computed tomography (CT) or magnetic resonance imaging (MRI) scan of the brain is usually warranted as part of the initial work-up, primarily to detect patterns of brain atrophy, and to evaluate for cerebrovascular disease. An MRI scan is helpful in looking for stroke. A CT scan is preferable over an MRI scan if the patient is falling and may have a possible subdural hematoma, if normal pressure hydrocephalus is being considered (with the triad of ataxia, confusion, and urinary incontinence), or if the patient has a pacemaker and is therefore not able to have an MRI scan. There are occasional instances in which a single photon emission computed tomography (SPECT) or positron emission tomography (PET) scan is useful in determining the type of dementia, most commonly in an effort to differentiate frontotemporal dementia versus early-stage Alzheimer's dementia.

More specialized testing may be needed and is guided by the clinician's suspicions of a specific disorder, e.g., seizures, meningitis, or toxic encephalopathy. If the patient has been acting out sexually, HIV testing and other sexually tranmitted disease (STD) screens should be ordered. Other examples of non-routine testing are electroencephalogram (EEG), which is useful with suspected seizure disorder or differentiating between dementia and delirium; heavy metal screening, copper and ceruloplasmin (for Wilson's disease), lumbar puncture, and/or blood cultures. A general principle here is that the work-up should be more extensive with early-onset dementia, as there is a greater chance of picking up uncommon or reversible pathology.

What is the role of consultants for inpatients with dementia?

General medical consultation and the availability of general medical coverage are of critical importance in taking care of patients with dementia on the psychiatric unit. Most often involved will be general internal medicine or geriatric medicine, cardiology, and neurology. In the elderly age group, psychiatric disorders and dementia are often accompanied by various and multiple medical co-morbidities, such as diabetes, hypertension, and chronic obstructive pulmonary disease. When physical examination and laboratory findings are pursued vigorously, psychiatric units have often been the site of first diagnosis of various general medical illnesses in this population; it is not unusual to discover parathyroid adenomas, normal pressure hydrocephalus, brain tumors, aspiration pneumonias, sepsis, hyponatremia, and other conditions on the psychiatric unit.

Neuropsychological testing can be useful in defining, quantifying, and localizing deficits in dementia. Physical therapy assessment and treatment on the unit are often necessary with the dementia population. Finally, an occupational therapy assessment of functioning can be an extremely important part of the evaluation – instrumental in deciding whether a patient can safely return home [12–14]. In the authors' experience, this information is also very helpful in convincing family members who feel guilty about putting their loved one "in a home" that they are making the best decision for the patient.

How important is it to distinguish the various forms of dementia?

Determining the precise diagnosis of a demented patient has utmost importance when a general medical or neurological condition that is potentially reversible presents as dementia. But even in the less dramatic cases, clinicians should categorize a patient's dementia as specifically as possible. The common groupings are Alzheimer's dementia, vascular dementia (formerly called multi-infarct dementia), Lewy body dementia (a.k.a. dementia with Lewy bodies, a.k.a. DLB), Wernicke–Korsakoff syndrome or other alcohol-related dementias, Huntington's chorea, frontotemporal dementia, and dementia related to Parkinson's disease (Tables 5.2 and 5.3). Patients within each of the various categories will exhibit different patterns of deficits, and will have different prognoses, treatment needs, and responses to medications. For instance, patients with Lewy body dementia are exquisitely sensitive to antipsychotic medications and can develop severe extra-pyramidal symptoms (EPS) or even neuroleptic malignant syndrome (NMS) in response to them. Quetiapine or

Table 5.2 Common dementia types and their characteristics

Alzheimer's dementia	40 to 60% of all dementias
	plaques and neurofibrillary tangles on histology
Parkinson's dementia	pre-existing history of the motor findings of Parkinson's disease
	occurs in 20 to 30% of Parkinson's patients
	tends to be a mild dementia
Dementia associated with Huntington's disease	genetic illness with trinucleotide (CAG) repeats
	onset in young or middle-aged adults
	choreiform movements
Frontotemporal dementia	prominent language deficits
	personality changes
	disinhibition
	executive functioning deficits
Lewy body dementia	Parkinsonian features
	visual hallucinations
	fluctuating cognitive deficits
	hypersensitivity to antipsychotics
Vascular (multi-infarct) dementia	step-wise decline in functioning
	history and other signs of atherosclerosis

clozapine, with relatively low incidence of EPS, would be the best choices if an antipsychotic is necessary for a patient with Lewy body dementia [15, 16]. Likewise, patients with Parkinson's dementias will be vulnerable to movement disorders with many of the antipsychotic medications and selective serotonin reuptake inhibitors (SSRIs), and thus treatment of psychosis and depression in these patients is quite a challenge. General guidelines for dementia related to Parkinson's would be to avoid high-potency traditional antipsychotics, avoid risperidone at dosages greater than 1 mg per day, and to consider a tricyclic antidepressant (TCA) or electroconvulsive therapy (ECT) for severe depression. (Treatment by ECT often makes the Parkinson's better, too.) Dementia of the Alzheimer's type is most likely to respond to cholinesterase inhibitors (donepezil, galantamine, rivastigmine) and N-methyl-D-aspartic acid (NMDA) receptor antagonists (memantine). Vascular dementia may require platelet aggregation inhibitors, anticoagulants, and better control of blood pressure [17].

Table 5.3 Distinguishing Alzheimer's dementia from frontotemporal dementia [21, 22]

Alzheimer's dementia	Frontotemporal dementia
Incidence increases with age	Onset at 35 to 75 years old, rare after age 75
Maintain social behavior in early stages	Early appearance of behavioral symptoms
Apathy when confused due to cognitive impairment	Pervasive apathy reflecting true motivational impairment
Early memory loss	Memory loss less prominent in early stages
Language dysfunction can occur as isolated cognitive feature	Language problems usually associated with memory loss
Spatial problems late in course	Spatial impairment earlier in course
Neuropsychological testing with more impairment of memory than executive tasks	Neuropsychological testing with more impairment in executive functioning than in memory

Refining the dementia diagnosis may be important to family members, who would likely be interested in their own genetic vulnerability to one of the types of dementia for which there is an understanding of the genetics. This includes Alzheimer's dementia, Huntington's dementia, and vascular dementia. At-risk relatives can pro-actively institute dietary, exercise, or even cognitive prophylaxis programs for themselves to reduce risk.

Ferreting out the possibility of dementia associated with alcohol dependence is necessary, as alcohol-related dementia and Korsakoff's dementia may improve to some extent with abstinence from alcohol and thiamine supplements [18, 19]. Of course, these patients are also at risk for alcohol withdrawal states upon admission if their dependence is not recognized and treated. Occasionally persons with eating disorders or malabsorption syndromes can also develop Wernicke–Korsakoff syndrome [19, 20]. For Wernicke's syndrome, the clinician should be alert to the constellation of delirium, ataxia, ophthalmoplegia, and lateral gaze nystagmus, though all three symptoms are only observed simultaneously in about one-fifth of cases [19].

How does one diagnose and treat depression in a patient with dementia?

Depression and dementia have a complicated relationship [23]. When they co-occur, depression can worsen cognition and cause a pre-existing dementia to appear more severe. Depression can also cause cognitive impairment, so-called pseudodementia, in people who are otherwise intact. Pseudodementia clears with improvement in mood. Finally, dementia can present with such severe affective blunting that one may wrongly diagnose a patient as depressed. Typically, the elderly patient with major depression will appear slowed and withdrawn and will make little effort to answer questions, while the purely demented patient will be more forthcoming, though evasive and confabulatory. Patients with dementia can also present with a co-occurring psychotic depression, diagnosis of which can be challenging due to overlap with dementia with psychotic features.

When patients have both depression and dementia, the depressive symptoms should be treated first. The clinician should find out what medications the patient has already tried, including the dosage and duration of any medication trials. Electroconvulsive therapy should always be considered, as it is often quicker and safer than medications. This is especially true in life or death situations, such as when patients are not eating/drinking or are seriously suicidal. When the diagnosis of psychotic depression is strongly suspected, ECT should be considered as the first-line option. One must keep in mind that ECT can cause cognitive impairment as a side effect. In a patient with mild dementia and severe depression who is receiving ECT, it is exceedingly important to track cognitive performance very closely [24, 25].

Selective serotonin reuptake inhibitors are generally the drugs of choice for depression in Alzheimer's patients. Among the SSRIs, those with more anticholinergic effect, such as paroxetine, are best avoided. Many geropsychiatrists prefer citalopram, escitalopram, or sertraline because of their relative lack of interactions with other medications [26]. Selective serotonin reuptake inhibitors can disrupt sleep, exacerbate or lead to movement disorders, and also have some risk of prolonging bleeding time. Mirtazapine is an appropriate alternative to the SSRIs, and is useful for patients who require sleep induction or appetite stimulation [27].

What is the best pharmacologic approach to dementia-related agitation?

Agitation is a common concomitant of the psychotic features that occur frequently in many forms of dementia. Severely agitated patients with dementia need to be calmed quickly upon admission to the unit. Various classes of medication can be used for this purpose [28–30]. Managing agitation in dementia requires both creativity and patience on the part of the psychiatrist, as elderly demented patients are highly variable in their responses, and are extremely susceptible to side effects (Table 5.4).

As with schizophrenia and mania, dementia with acute agitation can be treated with intramuscular (IM) or oral medications. Some patients may respond to a benzodiazepine alone, e.g., lorazepam 0.5 to 1 mg orally or IM. Intramuscular ziprasidone (10 mg initially followed by 10 mg twice daily as necessary) or IM olanzapine (2.5 to 5 mg as needed) can also be useful if the

Table 5.4 Medications that have been used for dementia-related agitation and/or psychosis [30]

Medication	Comments
Typical antipsychotics	helpful with paranoia, hallucinations, hostility, and agitation
	avoid with Parkinson's dementia and Lewy body dementia
	black-box warning
Atypical antipsychotics	first-line for paranoia, hallucinations, hostility, and aggression/agitation
	consider clozapine or quetiapine with DLB or Parkinson's dementia
	black-box warning
Antidepressants	not only for depression, but also agitation/irritability
	consider trazodone if sedation needed
	SSRIs preferable over TCAs
Anticonvulsants	for disruptive behavior, agitation, and sleep disturbance
	latest reviews suggest valproate side effects out-weigh benefits
Beta-blockers	limited support for efficacy with aggression, agitation, and anxiety
	frequent contraindications, some patients unable to tolerate

patient will not take oral medications. Haloperidol, alone or in combination with lorazepam, is still in common usage for agitated dementia patients. With the use of haloperidol, it is important to keep in mind that some dementias show particular sensitivity to traditional antipsychotics, with risk of development of serious EPS, catatonia, or NMS. A conservative approach involves starting at low doses in the elderly, as it may not require more than 0.25 to 0.5 mg of haloperidol twice daily to achieve control without side effects.

There is often pressure on the inpatient psychiatrist to eradicate psychotic symptoms and decrease associated behavioral disturbances. These are quite distressing to family members and caregivers, and might jeopardize the patient's ability to remain at home or to be managed adequately at an ECF. Anger, aggression, and paranoid ideas are symptoms that are particularly responsive to atypicals [31]. Two atypical antipsychotics that have been used extensively for dementia-related psychosis are risperidone, at a low starting dose such as 0.25 mg per day, and quetiapine, starting at 25 to 50 mg at bedtime. Both can be given in low doses during the day as necessary for breakthrough symptoms [32].

In 2005, a black-box warning was issued for the entire class of atypical antipsychotics when used for dementia-related psychosis, as a result of the discovery that these agents are associated with an increase in all-cause mortality rate by a factor of approximately 1.6 to 1.7 [28, 33]. More recent studies have shown that similar, if not greater, risk is attached to the use of traditional antipsychotics in dementia patients, and labels for these drugs are now also required to carry the warning [34]. These warnings have led most clinicians to be more cautious in use of both typical and atypical antipsychotics in dementia, and to consider use of behavioral interventions and other pharmacologic agents as alternatives to antipsychotics. But the clinical reality in some cases is that a patient will not be allowed to return to their home or the facility from which they came unless the inpatient psychiatry team gets behaviors under control as effectively and quickly as possible. So, even if the medications are necessary in these situations, at the very least, this statistical mortality data should lead clinicians to carefully document the rationale for their use and to obtain clear informed consent.

Anticonvulsants also may be effective for agitation in patients with dementia, especially carbamazepine, valproate, and oxcarbazepine [30]. Lithium can be used as well, initiated at a very low dose (e.g., 75 to 150 mg per day). Patients may respond at lithium blood levels in the range of 0.4 mEq/L, lower than those required for bipolar disorder treatment. Many clinicians, it should be noted, avoid lithium in these elderly patients because of the dual risks of cognitive impairment and overall toxicity due to decreased renal function with age.

In some instances of dementia-related agitation, the cognitive enhancers may be useful, even after the initial period of improvement that they afford for cognitive deficits. Selective serotonin reuptake inhibitors may also play a role in stemming agitation, even in the absence of significant depressive signs [35]. Trazodone can be used at bedtime for sedation, or in low doses throughout the day for its calming effects. Elderly dementia patients on trazodone should be monitored carefully for hypotension [36].

One relatively rare but dramatic situation faced on the inpatient psychiatric unit is the sexually inappropriate or sexually aggressive male patient. These patients are often younger, with frontotemporal dementia [37]. Selective serotonin reuptake inhibitors can be used for their libido-lowering effect. Rarely, chemical castration with conjugated estrogens or injectable medroxyprogesterone may be necessary to achieve control over this behavior [38, 39]. However, these drastic steps may not be necessary if non-pharmacologic measures, such as behavioral controls or sequestering the patient away from potential victims, are implemented.

In formulating a pharmacologic plan for the dementia patient, the physician should be guided by a focus on the patient's quality of life. For instance, medications may make the difference between a patient remaining at home and needing placement in a facility. As a general rule, patients who are ill

Table 5.5 *In our experience*. . . Hints for taking care of patients with dementia and agitation

Confirm that the referring providers or facility agree to accept the patient back after stabilization. Sad to say, but sometimes patients are "dumped" in the hospital emergency department.

Use medications if necessary, but remember that some degree of sedation, or other side effects, may be the price of control of agitation.

Family members need education about the limitations of psychopharmacology.

Keep in mind how taxing it can be for nursing staff to care for agitated demented patients. These patients can cause physical injury to staff.

Be constantly alert for medical/physical problems that lead to agitation in these patients.

Be aware of conflicting allegiances you may feel in caring for these patients. Who are you really treating? The referring facility, the family, or the patient?

Helping a dementia patient with psychosis/agitation can allow the patient to remain at home or in a less structured environment. This may represent a considerable success.

Remember: Patients with dementia-related agitation can be helped. . . with patience and teamwork

enough to require an inpatient hospitalization are likely ill enough to require a combination of psychotropic medications. It is not unusual to have to add and/ or subtract medications from the regimen during a hospitalization. Accurate nursing records of the patient's most agitated periods will help the psychiatrist design an efficacious dosing schedule of medication.

What other interventions can be helpful for psychiatric inpatients with dementia?

On the psychiatric unit, medication for dementia patients with agitation should be combined with strong behavioral approaches consisting of reality orientation, environmental manipulation, and close monitoring, sometimes even on a one-to-one basis. Staff should strive to create a calm setting for the patient, free of excessive environmental stimuli. Admittedly, this may be hard to achieve on a general psychiatric unit that serves patients who are young and patients who are elderly, those who are manic and those who are depressed. But efforts can be made to insulate patients with dementia from a busy milieu, for example, with age- or diagnosis-specific daily programming. Groups and activities for the inpatient with dementia can be tailored to the patient's cognitive level, with emphasis on engaging, but not over-stimulating, the patient. Reminiscence groups, music groups, and pet therapy may be particularly well received by this population [30]. A board or sign in the patient's room with the date and the names of the treatment team members is helpful in orienting the patient on a daily basis, as are efforts to avoid frequent shifts of primary caregivers. Pictures of family members and other familiar objects, such as quilts, restore a feeling of familiarity that dementia patients find calming. (See Table 5.5.)

References

1. Gurland B. Epidemiology of psychiatric disorders. In: Sadavoy J, Jarvik L, Grossberg G & Meyers B eds., *Comprehensive Textbook of Geriatric Psychiatry*, 3rd edn. New York, London: W. W. Norton & Co., Inc.; 2004, pp. 13–14.

2. Conn D. Other Dementias and Mental Disorders Due to General Medical Conditions. In: Sadavoy J, Jarvik L, Grossberg G & Meyers B eds., *Comprehensive Textbook of Geriatric Psychiatry*, 3rd edn. New York, London: W. W. Norton & Co., Inc.; 2004, pp. 545–79.

3. Almberg B, Grafström M & Winblad B. Caring for a demented elderly person: burden and burnout among caregiving relatives. *Journal of Advanced Nursing*, **25**:1 (1997), 109–16.

4. Knopman D, Berg J, Thomas R *et al.* Nursing home placement is related to dementia progression: experience from a clinical trial. *Neurology*, **52**:4 (1999), 714.

5. Smith G E, O'Brien P C, Ivnik R J, Kokmen E & Tangalos E G. Prospective analysis of risk factors for nursing home placement of dementia patients. *Neurology*, **57**:8 (2001), 1467–73.

6. Kapp M. Legal issues in dementia. *International Journal of Risk and Safety in Medicine*, **20**:1 (2008), 91–103.

7. Folstein M F, Folstein S E & McHugh P R. "Mini-mental state". A practical method for grading the cognitive state of patients for the clinician. *Journal of Psychiatric Research*, **12**:3 (1975), 189–98.

8. Nasreddine Z S, Phillips N A, Bedirian V *et al.* The Montreal Cognitive Assessment, MoCA: a brief screening tool for mild cognitive impairment. *Journal of the American Geriatrics Society*, **53**:4 (2005), 695–9.

9. Feldman H H, Jacova C, Robillard A *et al.* Diagnosis and treatment of dementia: 2. Diagnosis. *Canadian Medical Association Journal*, **178**:7 (2008), 825–36.

10. Alagiakrishnan K & Wiens C A. An approach to drug induced delirium in the elderly. *Postgraduate Medical Journal*, **80**:945 (2004), 388–93.

11. Boyle L, Ismail M & Porsteinsson A. Chapter 10: The dementia work-up. In: Agronin M & Maletta G eds., *Principles and Practice of Geriatric Psychiatry.* Philadelphia: Lippincott Williams & Wilkins; 2004.

12. Baird A. Fine tuning recommendations for older adults with memory complaints: using the Independent Living Scales with the Dementia Rating Scale. *Clinical Neuropsychologist*, **20**:4 (2006), 649–61.

13. Moore D, Palmer B, Patterson T & Jeste D. A review of performance-based measures of functional living skills. *Journal of Psychiatric Research*, **41**:1–2 (2007), 97–118.

14. Skelton F, Kunik M, Regev T & Naik A. Determining if an older adult can make and execute decisions to live safely at home: a capacity assessment and intervention model. *Archives of Gerontology and Geriatrics*, **50**:3 (2010), 300–5.

15. Raskind M, Bonner L & Peskind E. Cognitive disorders. In: Blazer D, Steffens D & Busse E eds., *The American Psychiatric Publishing Textbook of Geriatric Psychiatry*, 3rd edn. Washington DC: American Psychiatric Publishing, Inc.; 2004, p. 220.

16. Weintraub D & Hurtig H I. Presentation and management of psychosis in Parkinson's disease and dementia with Lewy bodies. *American Journal of Psychiatry*, **164**:10 (2007), 1491–8.

17. Wolf P A, Clagett G P, Easton J D *et al*. Preventing ischemic stroke in patients with prior stroke and transient ischemic attack: a statement for healthcare professionals from the Stroke Council of the American Heart Association. *Stroke*, **30**:9 (1999), 1991–4.

18. Thomson A & Marshall E. The natural history and pathophysiology of Wernicke's encephalopathy and Korsakoff's psychosis. *Alcohol and Alcoholism*, **41**:2 (2006), 151.

19. Sechi G & Serra A. Wernicke's encephalopathy: new clinical settings and recent advances in diagnosis and management. *Lancet Neurology*, **6**:5 (2007), 442–55.

20. Lindboe C & Loberg E. Wernicke's encephalopathy in non-alcoholics. An autopsy study. *Journal of Neurological Science*, **90**:2 (1989), 125–9.

21. McKhann G M, Albert M S, Grossman M *et al*. Clinical and pathological diagnosis of frontotemporal dementia: report of the Work Group on Frontotemporal Dementia and Pick's Disease. *Archives of Neurology*, **58**:11 (2001), 1803–9.

22. Pachana N A, Boone K B, Miller B L, Cummings J L & Berman N. Comparison of neuropsychological functioning in Alzheimer's disease and frontotemporal dementia. *Journal of the International Neuropsychological Society*, **2**:6 (1996), 505–10.

23. Alexopoulos G. Late-life mood disorders. In: Sadavoy J, Jarvik L, Grossberg G & Meyers B eds., *Comprehensive Textbook of Geriatric Psychiatry.* New York: W. W. Norton & Co., Inc.; 2004, pp. 616–17.

24. Lee H & Lyketsos C. Depression in Alzheimer's disease: heterogeneity and related issues. *Biological Psychiatry*, **54**:3 (2003), 353–62.

25. Lyketsos C & Olin J. Depression in Alzheimer's disease: overview and treatment. *Biological Psychiatry*, **52**:3 (2002), 243–52.

26. Lyketsos C, DelCampo L, Steinberg M *et al*. Treating depression in Alzheimer disease: efficacy and safety of sertraline therapy, and the benefits of depression reduction: the DIADS. *Archives of General Psychiatry*, **60**:7 (2003), 737.

27. Raji M & Brady S. Mirtazapine for treatment of depression and comorbidities in Alzheimer disease. *Annals of Pharmacotherapy*, **35**:9 (2001), 1024.

28. Jeste D V, Blazer D, Casey D *et al.* ACNP White Paper: update on use of antipsychotic drugs in elderly persons with dementia. *Neuropsychopharmacology*, **33**:5 (2007), 957–70.

29. Kunik M E, Yudofsky S C, Silver J M & Hales R E. Pharmacologic approach to management of agitation associated with dementia. *Journal of Clinical Psychiatry*. **55** Suppl (1994), 13–17.

30. Sadavoy J, Lanctot K & Deb S. Management of behavioural and psychological symptoms of dementia and acquired brain injury. In: Tyrer P & Silk K eds., *Effective Treatments in Psychiatry*. Cambridge: Cambridge University Press; 2008, p. 190.

31. Sultzer D L, Davis S M, Tariot P N *et al.* Clinical symptom responses to atypical antipsychotic medications in Alzheimer's disease: Phase 1 outcomes from the CATIE-AD Effectiveness Trial. *American Journal of Psychiatry*, **165**:7 (2008), 844–54.

32. Schneider L S, Dagerman K & Insel P S. Efficacy and adverse effects of atypical antipsychotics for dementia: meta-analysis of randomized, placebo-controlled trials. *American Journal of Geriatric Psychiatry*, **14**:3 (2006), 191–210.

33. Schneider L, Dagerman K & Insel P. Risk of death with atypical antipsychotic drug treatment for dementia: meta-analysis of randomized placebo-controlled trials. *Journal of the American Medical Association*, **294**:15 (2005), 1934.

34. Wang P, Schneeweiss S, Avorn J *et al.* Risk of death in elderly users of conventional vs. atypical antipsychotic medications. *New England Journal of Medicine*, **353**:22 (2005), 2335.

35. Pollock B G, Mulsant B H, Rosen J *et al.* Comparison of citalopram, perphenazine, and placebo for the acute treatment of psychosis and behavioral disturbances in hospitalized, demented patients. *American Journal of Psychiatry*, **159**:3 (2002), 460–5.

36. Sultzer D L, Gray K F, Gunay I, Berisford M A & Mahler M E. A double-blind comparison of trazodone and haloperidol for treatment of agitation in patients with dementia. *American Journal of Geriatric Psychiatry*, **5**:1 (1997), 60–9.

37. Miller B, Darby A, Benson D, Cummings J & Miller M. Aggressive, socially disruptive and antisocial behaviour associated with fronto-temporal dementia. *British Journal of Psychiatry*, **170**:2 (1997), 150.

38. Haussermann P, Goecker D, Beier K & Schroeder S. Low-dose cyproterone acetate treatment of sexual acting out in men with dementia. *International Psychogeriatrics*, **15**:2 (2003), 181–6.

39. Light S A & Holroyd S. The use of medroxyprogesterone acetate for the treatment of sexually inappropriate behaviour in patients with dementia. *Journal of Psychiatry & Neuroscience*, **31**:2 (2006), 132–4.

The inpatient with traumatic brain injury

When specific diagnoses are mentioned, we are referring to diagnoses and criteria as listed in the *Diagnostic and Statistical Manual of Mental Disorders*, 4th edition, text revision (DSM-IV-TR) unless otherwise specified.

What is the relevance of traumatic brain injury to psychiatric inpatient work?

In recent years, inpatient psychiatrists have become increasingly adept at recognizing and treating patients with neuropsychiatric sequelae of traumatic brain injury (TBI) [1–5]. In addition to the commonly seen TBI-related cognitive impairment, which is not the focus of this chapter, many post-TBI patients display atypical forms of mood and anxiety disorders, or even present with personality alterations and/or signs of behavioral dysregulation. Less frequently, long-term effects of TBI include various forms of psychosis, including delusions with persecutory content, and visual or auditory hallucinations. Expertise in recognition and management of TBI is made even more crucial by the increasing incidence of brain injuries in society, with U.S. emergency departments treating 444 new TBI cases per 100,000 people [6]. Traumatic brain injury occurs both in civilian life, resulting from motor vehicle accidents, violence, falls, and contact sports; and in the military, where penetrating and blast injuries are common causes [4, 7].

In the early stage of a moderate-to-severe TBI, patients are usually in encephalopathic states that can last days to months. Newly injured and sub-acute TBI patients are generally treated on surgical units or rehabilitation units while they are recovering from the initial injury. Sub-acute TBI patients will have regained consciousness, but are commonly agitated and delirious. Disoriented and disinhibited, TBI patients in early stages of recovery can be difficult to manage without one-to-one nursing care. During this period, TBI patients can easily become over-stimulated and may require treatment for the agitation. Although patients with TBI *can* become *more* disoriented with benzodiazepines, this class of medication is sometimes used for acute agitation. Some experts believe that in the very acute stages of TBI, antipsychotics, especially typical antipsychotics, should be avoided since dopamine D2 blockade can trigger cell death through glutamate cascades, thereby furthering the TBI damage [8].

With these early-stage TBI patients, the neurosurgical or rehabilitation teams are more likely to request psychiatric consultation/liaison input rather than psychiatric unit admission for the patient. By the intermediate phase, though, most of the acute manifestations of the injury are quieting down as the brain enters the next stage of recovery. In the intermediate stage the delirium/disorganization is resolving and patients progress toward more chronic neuropsychiatric syndromes, including behavioral/personality disturbances, affective dysregulation, and cognitive distortions/paranoia [4]. During this period, some patients enter long-term head injury rehabilitation facilities, where they can begin physical therapy, speech therapy, cognitive rehabilitation, and other physical medicine/rehabilitation modalities. The occasional TBI patient who is too aggressive to be handled at such a facility may be referred for inpatient psychiatric treatment and stabilization.

Six months to a year after the acute injury, the chronic or late effects of TBI emerge as "stable deficit" TBI-related neuropsychiatric disorders [9, 10]. The syndrome seen will depend upon the area of the brain that was damaged, the extent of damage, and the age of the patient, with older patients doing less well than younger patients. In terms of location of injury, frontal lobe injuries are associated with enduring defects in memory and executive functioning, and may present with problems in self-regulation. In contrast, temporal lobe involvement in TBI can lead to mania and psychosis as part of a temporal lobe epilepsy syndrome, or can result in affective symptoms or psychosis without associated seizures [11].

Given the strict criteria for psychiatric inpatient admission, it is likely that one large group of TBI patients warranting a stay on the psychiatric unit will be those who have threatened to harm themselves or others. These patients will likely fit into one of the affective-disordered, paranoid/psychotic, or disinhibited categories described with TBI. For some patients, the significance of a previously undiagnosed TBI – either as the sole cause of symptoms or as a contributing factor – is recognized for the first time on an inpatient psychiatry unit. One study of 100 psychiatric inpatients found a 68% prevalence of TBI, but no mention of the injuries in the psychiatric documentation [12]. All patients admitted with mood disorders or psychosis should be questioned about past head trauma.

Another group of patients admitted to inpatient psychiatric units will be from the one-third of patients with *mild* TBI who do not fully recover, but either languish in outpatient care, or without treatment at all. These patients have vague symptoms, including headaches, dizziness, sleep disturbance, and cognitive impairment, as well as anxiety and mood disturbance [13, 14]. This post-concussive syndrome can mimic various anxiety disorders and non-melancholic depression. The symptoms associated with a mild TBI are often subtle; patients can go years before clinicians associate their symptoms with a past history of a head injury or concussion. In addition, when mild TBI accompanies a pre-injury primary psychiatric disorder, patients have more frequent admission and longer stays on the inpatient unit than patients without TBI [15].

Lastly, TBI patients may benefit from an inpatient stay when they have deficient coping skills, and are reacting to the injury with feelings of hopelessness, overwhelming anxiety, or behavioral regression. These patients may have sub-threshold post-traumatic stress disorder (PTSD) symptoms or even frank PTSD [9]. Traumatic brain injury patients with pre-morbid histories of abuse may be particularly vulnerable to psychologically traumatic aspects of TBI [16].

What happens to the brain in TBI that leads to psychiatric problems?

In brain injuries, a combination of neuroanatomical and neurochemical disruptions contributes to disturbances in normal functioning [3, 4]. There are a number of neurophysiologic mechanisms that lead to TBI, including penetrative injuries with tissue disruption, compression injuries, such as those occurring secondary to subdural hematomas or other bleeds, and shearing force trauma [9, 17]. Shearing force trauma is associated with acceleration–deceleration and rotational forces, and can lead to axonal injury via stretching of axons. Other mechanical factors can be prominent when brain matter stretches over rough surfaces, such as that of the sphenoid bone. Secondary TBI injury mechanisms include brain edema, hypoxia secondary to cerebral perfusion pressure, and neuronal damage and cytochemical disruption caused by release of excitatory neurotransmitters from injured neurons [14]. When the head is stationary, as in a blow to the head, the injury is typically under the site of impact. When the head is in motion, as in a fall or auto accident, the torsion injury is termed "coup-contrecoup" and opposite sides of the brain can be injured at the same time [2, 18]. In TBI, partial recovery of overall functioning is aided by the brain's extensive connectivity. However, there are limits to this mending because of neuronal cell body death. Most meaningful recovery occurs within 12 to 18 months after the initial injury. In the later stages of TBI recovery, gliosis occurs, which can be a cause of later-occurring seizure disorders [11].

How does one measure the severity of a TBI?

The Glasgow Coma Scale (GCS), assessed right after the injury, is an indirect measure of TBI severity [8]. The lowest score possible is 3 and the highest 15. A GCS of 13 to 15 is considered a mild TBI, equivalent to a concussion. Patients with mild injuries may only have dizziness and diplopia immediately following the event, but this can evolve into a headache and concentration problems that persist for weeks. A moderate TBI correlates with a GCS of 9 to 12, while a severe TBI scores 8 or less. The duration of loss of consciousness (LOC) is another measure of the severity of TBI; where mild TBI has a LOC of less than 20 minutes, moderate TBI between 20 and 60 minutes, and severe TBI greater than 60 minutes. Yet another indicator of the severity of TBI is the extent of post-traumatic amnesia. For instance, two weeks of amnesia would generally be associated with severe TBI.

Assessing severity is important, since that also has predictive value regarding the likelihood of psychiatric sequelae. Taylor lists what kinds of TBI are usually significant enough to contribute to or cause psychiatric conditions later on [11]:

all open head injuries; and

closed head injuries with one (or more) of the following:

15 minutes (or more) of unconsciousness

skull fracture or intracranial hemorrhage

focal neurological signs at the time of the injury

seizure at the time of the injury

noticeable period of anterograde amnesia following injury

prolonged poor functioning post-injury.

What pre-morbid factors influence a TBI patient's presentation and ultimate prognosis?

A brain injury is not only a physical event, but also a psychologically devastating incident in the life of a unique person. Therefore the soundness of the pre-TBI "self" is an important determinant of the success of rehabilitative treatment and the ultimate outcome of the injury. The patient's unique set of coping mechanisms, personality traits, and pre-morbid psychiatric vulnerabilities will come into play in dealing with the multiple stressors inherent in a TBI, which include the impact on appearance, cognitive functioning, job performance, and interpersonal relationships [9]. Although there is a correlation between the extent of injury and the occurrence/severity of psychiatric manifestations, any pre-morbid pathology – be it a mood disorder or personality traits – has a major effect on clinical presentation after the TBI [19].

Pre-morbid diagnoses of a TBI patient may also include a substance use disorder. One study of "new" TBI patients found incidences of "at risk" drinking and illicit drug use of 59% and 34% respectively [20]. Not surprisingly, alcohol is implicated in a large percentage of the TBIs related to motor vehicle accidents. Furthermore, a history of previous TBI renders patients more susceptible to further head injuries (i.e., a TBI is a risk factor for another TBI). The psychosocial situation of the patient could limit or enhance the subsequent treatment approach to a particular patient's TBI syndrome. For example, the treatment team will need to take into account the impact of the TBI on the patient's pre-existing support network of family, friends, and faith community.

It is not uncommon for TBI patients to lose support by alienating others with provocative behaviors.

What are the elements of a good TBI evaluation on the inpatient unit?

If TBI is suspected or known, patients should have the standard inpatient evaluation with added attention to the possibility of a TBI-related syndrome. History of the accident itself should be gathered, including type of accident, period of loss of consciousness, any report of scales used in the acute phase, and history of subdural hematoma, surgeries, seizures, etc. It is useful to review any previous reports and imaging studies, with attention to localization of the injury. Shearing-force damage may be seen on a magnetic resonance imaging (MRI) scan as multiple focal lesions throughout the white matter, but sometimes it is not visible at all. In general, with TBI, MRI scan is preferable to computed tomography (CT) scan as scarring will show up more readily. And, as mentioned above, past psychiatric history is important since TBI can exacerbate pre-existing illnesses.

Family interviews may be necessary due to the patient's injury-related amnesia for events around the actual accident, or because current lack of insight might hamper the ability to accurately report the extent of TBI-related symptoms [21]. The family psychiatric history is also important as TBI may unmask a heretofore unexpressed genotype. Neuropsychiatric testing can assist with more precise determination of the pattern of deficits. By the time a patient arrives on an inpatient unit they probably already have had multiple laboratory tests. Tests for treatable causes of brain disease – including thyroid functions, VDRL (Venereal Disease Research Laboratory) test, ANA (antinuclear antibody) test, vitamin B12, toxicology, and urine drug screening – should be reviewed or completed.

Other issues to consider include pre-morbid functioning, presence of pre-injury Axis II disorders or traits, and pre-morbid substance use. Many of these patients will be on a polypharmacy regimen that may already include psychotropics and opiate pain medications. Therefore, treating clinicians need to pay close attention to possible drug–drug interactions and to medication side effects masquerading as psychiatric symptoms.

What are the common TBI-related syndromes treated on the inpatient unit?

Mood disorders are common in TBI, with depression occurring in up to 50% of patients [22]. Depressive symptoms may be correlated with damage to frontal–parietal areas, and can occur at any time in the course of recovery from TBI. Despite some correlations with functional neuroanatomy, depression in TBI is probably best understood from a biopsychosocial perspective, with multi-factorial contributions to the mood disturbance [4]. Furthermore, TBI-related depression has a significant suicide rate, 15 to 20%, and thus needs to be treated aggressively [23]. Post-TBI mania occurs less commonly, in less than 10% of cases, either as an unmasking of pre-TBI bipolar disorder or arising de novo from the injury [1, 24].

The most common TBI-associated psychotic states are paranoid in nature. These are difficult to treat as the patients often seem cognitively "frozen" in their paranoid projections and lack mentalization skills to reflect on their symptoms. These states can range from querulous and suspicious to frankly delusional [25]. Anxiety states related to TBI can resemble generalized anxiety disorder or panic disorder. They can also take the form of PTSD-like states related to the initial accident situation [26].

Aggressive states and irritability are common sequelae of TBI, and indeed are often the cause of hospital admission [27]. These patients show very little ability to tolerate stimuli. They "go off" on others quickly, with minor provocation, and often show signs of paranoia as well. In some respects, these patients resemble patients with DSM-IV-TR personality disorders but with a greater degree of impulsivity/disinhibition, hyper-emotionality, and lability. These "externalizing" symptoms are thought to be related to damage in regions of the orbitofrontal cortex, anterior temporal lobe cortex, the amygdala, and the connecting circuits between those areas [28]. A TBI-related frontal lobe syndrome can also present with flatness of mood, lack of social graces and empathy, and decreased attention to self-care [29].

How common is malingering or exaggeration of TBI-related complaints?

Though much has been written about litigation and secondary gain with head injuries, malingering is actually not common [30]. Secondary gain is often wrongfully suspected because the psychiatric manifestations of TBI can be present long after the physical and neurological signs have stabilized or abated. In addition, many health care providers have difficulty accepting that a mild TBI can be associated with more severe lasting neuropsychiatric impairment [31]. Research into TBI has found that the initial severity of illness is not necessarily correlated with the severity of a subsequent post-TBI neuropsychiatric syndrome [32].

What are the pros and cons of admitting TBI patients to a psychiatric unit?

The hospital can provide a safe environment for observation and treatment of TBI patients. Staff can observe their everyday functioning and closely monitor the response to various pharmacologic trials. Family members, who may become frustrated when the physical aspects of the TBI are improving while

Table 6.1 Tips for behavioral management of patients with TBI [33]

Consistent staffing is best; TBI patients do not react well to changes
Tailor expectations in groups and activities to the TBI patient's capabilities, thereby allowing the patient to avoid frustration and to have self-esteem enhancing successes
Allow the patient some control and meaningful choices whenever possible
Avoid surprises by carefully preparing the patient for any new approaches, medications, blood draws, and other tests
Regular daily routine is important, including some kind of visual display of the schedule and staff names
Employ re-direction, diversion, and "time outs" for negative behaviors
Identify and address triggers to negative behaviors, e.g., stressful visits from family, response to limit setting, interactions with other patients

the emotional symptoms are still persistent, can benefit from the respite offered by a hospital stay. Patients with TBI often exhibit significant self-loathing and can thus benefit from inpatient groups and activities that are directed at allowing mourning the lost "pre-TBI self" while building new coping skills.

These are not easy patients. Staff may struggle to handle the special demands of the TBI patient, including the ever-present risk of aggressive acting out. Traumatic brain injury patients can potentially be disruptive to the therapeutic milieu, and may not fit comfortably with the majority of routine psychiatric patients found on a general psychiatric unit. Staff's familiarity and skill at behavioral interventions for TBI patients is necessary, as these techniques have been shown to be effective adjuncts to pharmacotherapy for TBI patients with agitation, irritability, and other signs of emotional dyscontrol (Table 6.1) [28]. Often these patients require one-to-one staffing. The families of TBI patients are often in turmoil as well and require more than the usual amount of social work attention. Patients with TBI may have prolonged stays on the unit, due in part to the complicated nature of their presentations, and because medication "up-titrations" must proceed slowly due to heightened sensitivity to medication side effects. Productive team meetings and strong leadership are essential if the hospitalization is to be successful.

Which medications are helpful in managing TBI-related psychiatric symptoms?

Despite ample studies of the efficacy of various agents for TBI-related symptoms, there are currently no medications that have been FDA-approved for TBI, and use is therefore "off-label" (Table 6.2). Useful reviews on this topic,

Table 6.2 Medications for TBI-related neuropsychiatric syndromes/symptoms

Medication	Comments
Beta-blockers (e.g., propranolol)	useful for outbursts/aggression
	high doses may be necessary
Benzodiazepines	for agitation
	sedation or paradoxical reactions may be problematic
	short-term use only recommended
TCAs	more side effects than SSRIs in depressive syndromes
	may help with chronic pain
Amantadine	good effects on cognition and aggression for some patients
SSRIs and SNRIs	treat depressive symptoms and agitation,
	citalopram has best evidence
Buspirone	useful when agitation is related to underlying anxiety
	slow onset of action
Trazodone	may be useful for agitation/aggression
	can help with sleep
	fewer side effects than antipsychotics
Anticonvulsants (e.g., valproate, carbamazepine, and lamotrigine	for agitation, aggression, affective instability
	best evidence for carbamazepine
Lithium	some anti-aggressive effects
	mixed reports of efficacy in TBI
	best use for patients with pre-morbid bipolar disorder
	watch for neurotoxic effects/confusion
Antipsychotics	superior to placebo for agitation
	best use for patients with associated paranoia/psychosis
	atypicals with less EPS than typicals
Psychostimulants (e.g., methylphenidate)	for patients with problems in arousal, attention, and motivation
Hormonal agents (e.g., estrogen and medroxyprogesterone)	reports of reduction in hypersexual aggressive behaviors

which were the foundational material for this section, have been written by Levy *et al.* [34], Siddall [35], Ripley [36], Lombard and Zafonte [37], Corrigan *et al.* [38], Kile *et al.* [39], and Zafonte *et al.* [40].

Propranolol has been used, with some success, to treat aggression in TBI. A starting dose of 20 mg three times daily, with increases every 3 to 5 days to a maximum of 600 mg total per day, has been effective. Close monitoring of pulse, blood pressure, and electrocardiogram (EKG) is necessary as dosing increases. Amantadine has also been shown to have effects on aggression and cognition in TBI, with doses ranging from 50 to 400 mg per day. Brief use of benzodiazepines for severe agitation *may* be warranted, but regular use can lead to further disinhibition, and thus is not recommended. Lithium and the anticonvulsants – including carbamazepine, valproate, and lamotrigine – are useful for hypomania/mania, agitation, and irritability. Dosage ranges for these may be comparable to those used for bipolar disorders, with the caveat that the injured brain is much more sensitive to the effects of these medications and dose titration needs to proceed gingerly. Antipsychotics, including both typicals and atypicals, have some place in treatment as well, especially in those patients with paranoia and delusions. The principle here, as with other medications for TBI, is to start with low doses and increase slowly. Some of the atypicals (i.e., ziprasidone and aripiprazole) tend to be activating in TBI. Caution is advised with their use. Clozapine is a last-resort agent for TBI-related aggression or psychosis. While a positive feature is clozapine's low incidence of extra-pyramidal symptoms (EPS), its association with increased risk of seizures presents a problem in TBI.

Disinhibited TBI patients may benefit from antipsychotics, mood stabilizers, lithium, or amantadine. Attention-deficit/hyperactivity disorder (ADHD) medications (e.g., stimulants and atomoxetine) are most helpful for TBI patients with difficulties in initiation and attention, but may also decrease angry outbursts in some patients.

Selective serotonin reuptake inhibitors (SSRIs) and/or serotonin and norepinephrine reuptake inhibitors (SNRIs) are useful for TBI-related depression, either alone or in combination with a mood stabilizer. Tricyclic antidepressants (TCAs) have also shown efficacy in depression with TBI. Though much of the initial literature on TCAs for TBI-related depression examined the efficacy of amitriptyline, secondary amines like desipramine or nortriptyline may be equally effective with less anticholinergic action, and are thus preferred. In patients where improved sleep is desired, trazodone or mirtazapine can be useful. Monoamine oxidase inhibitors (MAOIs) are less commonly employed but are still an option for some patients who are able to follow the dietary restrictions. Finally, although electroconvulsive therapy (ECT) is often not considered in the TBI patient because of the fear of worsening cognition, it can be used effectively and is especially indicated for psychotic depression in TBI.

For anxiety symptoms, SSRIs/SNRIs and mood stabilizers are preferable to benzodiazepines. However, clinicians need to be alert to the risk that SSRIs may cause agitation and over-activation, as well as dystonia, in patients with TBI. The TCAs or mirtazapine are less problematic in this regard. Benzodiazepines can be used in some TBI patients in the early stages of treatment if absolutely necessary, and can be supplemented by cognitive–behavioral therapy (CBT) with selected patients. But attempts should be made to transition to an SSRI, SNRI, or another agent.

Combinations of medications tend to be common in the treatment of TBI because of the complexity of TBI neuropsychiatric presentations and the frequency of a multi-symptom picture. Several caveats are important to remember with polypharmacy in TBI. Awareness of possible drug–drug interactions and possible neurotoxicity is key. Sequencing the addition of medications should focus first on alleviating the patient's agitation. Initial control of agitation often necessitates starting off with a mood stabilizer or antipsychotic. Furthermore, clinicians should not become so invested in finding the "magic bullet" of medications that non-biological contributions to agitation or depression are overlooked. If a given patient is not doing well on the psychiatric inpatient unit despite extensive trials of medications, the clinician should review what is happening with the patient on the unit, including interactions with staff and other patients, and possible stress from family visits.

How does one approach psychiatric inpatients with both TBI and substance use disorders?

When TBI is accompanied by substance use, a general rule is that it is essential to get patients off drugs and alcohol in order to treat the TBI-related psychiatric syndrome. Since TBI patients may be prone to develop a secondary substance use disorder, the clinician needs to be flexible and creative, but clinically aggressive in treating symptoms that are fostering the use of substances and alcohol. When TBI patients who are abusing substances arrive on the inpatient unit, they benefit from most aspects of substance treatment described elsewhere in this manual (see Chapter 7), with the reminder that motivational interviewing techniques may need to be modified to adjust to the cognitive limitations of some TBI patients. Interestingly, TBI is often missed as an etiologic factor in the development of a substance-use disorder and may be "discovered" for the first time on the inpatient unit. The treatment team should be willing to contend with the patient's psychosocial situation, and enlist family support to provide an external framework for recovery/abstinence. Overall, the best approach to the TBI patient with substance use is one that combines educational and modified motivational elements, involves both patient and family, and incorporates an attitude from the treatment team of "flexibility without indulgence." Even with all of that in place, these patients can be challenging to manage successfully. They may require referral to primary addiction treatment facilities once the TBI-related symptoms are stabilized on the psychiatric unit [38].

References

1. Kim E, Lauterbach E C, Reeve A *et al.* Neuropsychiatric complications of traumatic brain injury: a critical review of the literature (a report by the ANPA Committee on Research). *Journal of Neuropsychiatry & Clinical Neurosciences*, **19**:2 (2007), 106–127.

2. Nicholl J & LaFrance W Jr. Neuropsychiatric sequelae of traumatic brain injury. *Seminars in Neurology*, **29** (2009), 247.

3. Rao V & Lyketsos C. Neuropsychiatric sequelae of traumatic brain injury. *Psychosomatics*, **41**:2 (2000), 95–103.

4. Rao V & Lyketsos C G. Psychiatric aspects of traumatic brain injury. *Psychiatric Clinics of North America*, **25**:1 (2002), 43–69.

5. Warriner E M & Velikonja D. Psychiatric disturbances after traumatic brain injury: neurobehavioral and personality changes. *Current Psychiatry Reports*, **8**:1 (2006), 73–80.

6. Jager T E, Weiss H B, Coben J H & Pepe P E. Traumatic brain injuries evaluated in U.S. emergency departments, 1992–1994. *Academic Emergency Medicine*, **7**:2 (2000), 134–40.

7. Williams J. Serving the health needs of our military veterans. *North Carolina Medical Journal*, **69**:1 (2008), 23–6.

8. Silver J, Hales R & Yudofsky S. Neuropsychiatric aspects of traumatic brain injury. In: Yudofsky S & Hales R eds., *The American Psychiatric Publishing Textbook of Neuropsychiatry and Clinical Sciences.* Washington DC: American Psychiatric Publishing, Inc.; 2002.

9. Nicholl J & LaFrance W C Jr. Neuropsychiatric sequelae of traumatic brain injury. *Seminars in Neurology*, **29**:3 (2009), 247–55.

10. Deb S, Lyons I, Koutzoukis C, Ali I & McCarthy G. Rate of psychiatric illness 1 year after traumatic brain injury. *American Journal of Psychiatry*, **156**:3 (1999), 374.

11. Taylor M. Chapter 11: Traumatic brain injury and stroke. In: Taylor M ed., *The Fundamentals of Clinical Neuropsychiatry*, Oxford: Oxford University Press; 1999.

12. Burg J, McGuire L, Burright R & Donovick P. Prevalence of traumatic brain injury in an inpatient psychiatric population. *Journal of Clinical Psychology in Medical Settings*, **3**:3 (1996), 243–51.

13. Lishman W A. Physiogenesis and psychogenesis in the "post-concussional syndrome". *British Journal of Psychiatry*, **153**:4 (1988), 460–9.

14. Silver J M, McAllister T W & Arciniegas D B. Depression and cognitive complaints following mild traumatic brain injury. *American Journal of Psychiatry*, **166**:6 (2009), 653–61.

15. Mateo M A, Glod C A, Hennen J, Price B H & Merrill N. Mild traumatic brain injury in psychiatric inpatients. *Journal of Neuroscience Nursing*, **37**:1 (2005), 28–33.

16. Raskin S A. The relationship between sexual abuse and mild traumatic brain injury. *Brain Injury*, **11**:8 (1997), 587–603.

17. Ray S K, Dixon C E & Banik N L. Molecular mechanisms in the pathogenesis of traumatic brain injury. *Histology & Histopathology*, **17**:4 (2002), 1137–52.

18. Nicholl J, LaFrance W Jr. Neuropsychiatric sequelae of traumatic brain injury. *Seminars in Neurology*, **29**:3 (2009), 247–55

19. Rogers J M & Read C A. Psychiatric comorbidity following traumatic brain injury. *Brain Injury*, **21**:13 (2007), 1321–33.

20. Bombardier C H, Rimmele C T & Zintel H. The magnitude and correlates of alcohol and drug use before traumatic brain injury. *Archives of Physical Medicine & Rehabilitation*, **83**:12 (2002), 1765–73.

21. Bogod N, Mateer C & Macdonald S. Self-awareness after traumatic brain injury: a comparison of measures and their relationship to executive functions. *Journal of the International Neuropsychological Society*, **9**:3 (2003), 450–8.

22. Jorge R & Robinson R G. Mood disorders following traumatic brain injury. *Neurorehabilitation*, **17**:4 (2002), 311–24.

23. Teasdale T W & Engberg A W. Suicide after traumatic brain injury: a population study. *Journal of Neurology, Neurosurgery & Psychiatry*, **71**:4 (2001), 436–40.

24. Shukla S, Cook B, Mukherjee S, Godwin C & Miller M. Mania following head trauma. *American Journal of Psychiatry*, **144**:1 (1987), 93.

25. Zhang Q & Sachdev P S. Psychotic disorder and traumatic brain injury. *Current Psychiatry Reports*, **5**:3 (2003), 197–201.

26. Hiott D W & Labbate L. Anxiety disorders associated with traumatic brain injuries. *Neurorehabilitation*, **17**:4 (2002), 345–55.

27. Kim E. Agitation, aggression, and disinhibition syndromes after traumatic brain injury. *Neurorehabilitation*, **17**:4 (2002), 297–310.

28. Ylvisaker M, Turkstra L, Coehlo C *et al*. Behavioural interventions for children and adults with behaviour disorders after TBI: a systematic review of the evidence. *Brain Injury*, **21**:8 (2007), 769–805.

29. Kant R & Smith-Seemiller L. Assessment and treatment of apathy syndrome following head injury. *Neurorehabilitation*, **17**:4 (2002), 325–31.

30. Miller L. Not just malingering: syndrome diagnosis in traumatic brain injury litigation. *Neurorehabilitation*, **16**:2 (2001), 109–22.

31. Swift T L & Wilson S L. Misconceptions about brain injury among the general public and non-expert health professionals: an exploratory study. *Brain Injury*, **15**:2 (2001), 149–65.

32. van Reekum R, Cohen T & Wong J. Can traumatic brain injury cause psychiatric disorders? *Journal of Neuropsychiatry and Clinical Neurosciences*, **12**:3 (2000), 316.

33. Ylvisaker M, Turkstra L, Coehlo C *et al*. Behavioural interventions for children and adults with behaviour disorders after TBI: a systematic review of the evidence. *Brain Injury*, **21**:8 (2007), 769–805.

34. Levy M, Berson A, Cook T *et al.* Treatment of agitation following traumatic brain injury: a review of the literature. *Neurorehabilitation*, **20**:4 (2005), 279–306.

35. Siddall O R M. Use of methylphenidate in traumatic brain injury. *Annals of Pharmacotherapy*, **39**:7–8 (2005), 1309–13.

36. Ripley D L. Atomoxetine for individuals with traumatic brain injury. *Journal of Head Trauma Rehabilitation*, **21**:1 (2006), 85–8.

37. Lombard L A & Zafonte R D. Agitation after traumatic brain injury: considerations and treatment options. *American Journal of Physical Medicine & Rehabilitation*, **84**:10 (2005), 797–812.

38. Corrigan J D, Lamb-Hart G L & Rust E. A programme of intervention for substance use following traumatic brain injury. *Brain Injury*, **9**:3 (1995), 221–36.

39. Kile S, Bourgeois J, Sugden S *et al.* Neurobehavioral sequelae of traumatic brain injury. *Psychiatric Times*, **1** December 2005.

40. Zafonte R, Cullen N & Lexell J. Serotonin agents in the treatment of acquired brain injury. *Journal of Head Trauma Rehabilitation*, **17**:4 (2002), 322.

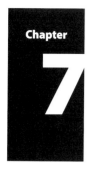

The inpatient with dual diagnosis

When specific diagnoses are mentioned, we are referring to diagnoses and criteria as listed in the *Diagnostic and Statistical Manual of Mental Disorders*, 4th edition, text revision (DSM-IV-TR) unless otherwise specified.

Why are patients with dual diagnosis disorders admitted to an inpatient psychiatric unit?

First, a clarification of vocabulary. In this volume the terms "dual diagnosis," "substance use disorder[s]," "[name of substance] use," and/or "[name of substance] dependence" are used. The first two, more general, terms are used more or less interchangeably, with recognition that a patient can have a substance use disorder (SUD) without having dual diagnosis – i.e., without a separate, primary psychiatric illness [1]. The assumption is made that, unless mentioned specifically, clinical situations discussed here involve patients who do have a primary psychiatric illness in addition to a SUD. Also, although DSM-IV criteria differentiate between substance abuse and substance dependence, this volume, again unless specifically mentioned, does not make that distinction. Furthermore, the authors avoid the term "substance abuse" altogether, given recent evidence that this phrase propagates stigma against a very large sub-set of the psychiatric patient population [2].

Similar to syphilis several generations ago, addiction is the modern "great imitator" of psychiatric symptoms and syndromes, as well as a frequent concomitant of psychiatric illness [3]. With psychiatric illness, dual diagnosis may be more the rule than the exception, with substance dependence tripling the odds of a psychiatric disorder, and psychiatric disorders similarly increasing the chances of a SUD [4]. This association has been found across psychiatric diagnoses, both in the United States and internationally [5]. Patients with either primary substance dependency or dual diagnosis can present to psychiatric emergency departments in psychotic, manic, depressed, or highly anxious states [6]. When these symptoms are severe – as is often the case – these patients are often admitted to psychiatric units, where their clinical state can be assessed, classified, monitored, and treated. In these instances, the inpatient unit becomes the site for determining whether the presenting symptoms have been induced by substance use alone or the substance use has uncovered/exacerbated symptoms of a primary psychiatric diagnosis [1].

Inpatient psychiatrists need to be mindful of the possible role of a substance use disorder throughout *any* patient's hospitalization, beginning with the evaluation itself and extending into the treatment phase and discharge planning. For example, if a patient is still intoxicated on admission, the evaluation may need to be delayed; a previously occult SUD may be discovered only when a patient experiences withdrawal several days into his/her stay; and follow-up for these patients should include treatment that will address the substance problem [7–10]. Information may come to light that leads the team to dispense with a primary psychiatric diagnosis, replacing it with a substance-induced mood, anxiety, or psychotic disorder diagnosis in the chart. Conversely, patients are admitted to the hospital with "history of substance-induced [blank] disorder" all through the chart when observation and investigation by the inpatient team reveals convincing evidence for addition of a primary Axis I disorder [11, 12].

It has been argued that psychiatrists are not well trained in recognizing and managing dual diagnosis disorders [13]. Clinicians in inpatient settings should acquire proficiency in recognition of SUDs in all patients. In addition, core competencies of inpatient psychiatry include management of withdrawal states, an understanding of the "disease model" of addiction, and an appreciation of psychosocial aspects of addiction.

The increasing prevalence of dual-diagnosis disorders requires close co-operation between inpatient psychiatric units and chemical dependency programs [14]. Occasionally patients with dual-diagnosis disorders begin treatment at a substance abuse facility and are subsequently transferred to a psychiatric hospital for intensive treatment of the psychiatric disorder. For example, a patient may begin detoxification in a substance treatment program and as the treatment proceeds, staff see underlying psychiatric symptoms that are too severe to be managed safely outside a psychiatric unit. Patients who are depressed and intensely suicidal, floridly manic, or severely psychotic are best served by management and stabilization on a psychiatric unit – with transfer back to the substance abuse center afterwards [15].

Virtually all abusable substances are associated with an increased risk of suicide [16–18]. But special considerations are needed when suicidal patients with SUD present with symptoms of intoxication or withdrawal; the severity or pattern of symptoms might necessitate a general medical or even intensive care unit (ICU) admission. More medically stable patients can be admitted directly to the psychiatric unit for treatment of the mood or psychotic symptoms.

What are the issues in SUDs that inpatient psychiatric clinicians often miss?

Clinicians need to remember that alcohol *is* a sedative-hypnotic drug. Thus, when patients are withdrawing from alcohol – even if they are psychotic from delirium tremens or from a primary psychotic disorder – they will require treatment with medication that has true sedative-hypnotic properties and cross-tolerance with alcohol in addition to medication for the psychosis. Antipsychotic medications have little affinity for the gamma-aminobutyric acid (GABA) receptor and by themselves are ineffective for withdrawal symptoms.

However, another problem is the *overuse* of benzodiazepines on psychiatric units, which is supported by multiple studies that 50 to 70% of psychiatric inpatients are prescribed sedatives, either scheduled or as needed [19, 20]. While benzodiazepines have a legitimate inpatient role for a number of disorders – including their place in detoxification – long-term use should be avoided in a patient with a dual diagnosis history [19].

Finally, even a seasoned psychiatrist may be fooled by patients with dual diagnosis or a primary SUD who are in denial of their addiction. Furthermore, the historical split between the fields of psychiatry and chemical dependency has fostered a certain disjointed quality to treatment of dual-diagnosis patients [21, 22]. This has made it more likely that a clinician focused on the primary psychiatric disorder will collude with the patient's defensiveness around chemical dependency. This split is being addressed through greater integration of the two areas, with an increase in medical education in addiction, and the development of specialized fellowships in addiction psychiatry [13, 14, 23, 24].

What are the important elements of the inpatient evaluation of dual diagnosis?

A brief case vignette illustrates how dual diagnosis may reveal itself in the course of an inpatient evaluation:

> For years, a 50-year-old internist had been writing prescriptions for opiates for himself. His opiate addiction came to light only after he was admitted in a serious manic state to a psychiatric unit. He gave the history that he had been followed by an outpatient psychiatrist who had been treating him with lithium and valproate for his mood disorder. He told the inpatient psychiatrist that he "had been praying" that his outpatient doctor would ask him about his opiate use or obtain a urine drug screen. As a physician himself, this patient had been too ashamed to bring up his addiction to the psychiatrist who "knew him best."

This all-too-common scenario highlights the guilt and shame commonly accompanying a SUD. To counteract the patient's negative self-evaluation, the clinician should create a non-judgmental interview situation in which substance use can be discussed in a matter-of-fact manner. Whether chemical dependency is suspected or has already been confirmed, the psychiatrist should strive to take an approach in which the addiction is treated like any other medical disorder. Psychiatrists who mix up the "patient" with the "addiction" can become critical, overly confrontational, and moralistic toward the patient with a SUD. Societal attitudes towards addiction can also divert the clinician from a neutral stance. A large percentage of the population still views chemical dependency as a moral or character failure.

When delving into the history of substance use, the interviewer will have better luck with a general assumption of use rather than with hesitant questions beginning with the phrase "have you ever used. . .?" The psychiatrist can start the inquiry with alcohol use, since it is usually more socially acceptable and not illegal, with a line of questioning beginning with first use, then progressing to peak use, regular use, and finally, last use. Thus the questions are:

> "How old were you when you first used alcohol?"
> "At your peak use, how much and how often were you drinking?"
> "At what age did you start using alcohol on a regular basis?"
> "When did you drink last?"

The same line of systematic questioning can then be applied for other substances, including nicotine, opiates, inhalants, hallucinogens, cannabis, amphetamines and cocaine. It is also important to ask the question "What prescription drugs have you overused or used when they were not prescribed to you?" When patients are overusing prescribed medications, it is important to determine how and why they were originally started – headaches, back pain, and post-surgery pain are common reasons – so that the clinician can begin to consider non-habit-forming alternatives. When asking about heroin and/or cocaine use, it is necessary to find out if the patient was snorting, shooting, or smoking the drug. Intravenous use, of course, has numerous medical implications.

Another element of the evaluation that has particular significance for addiction is a search for a history of trauma, losses, and abuse [25, 26]. Many patients with addictions have never revealed these historical elements to a professional, or indeed, to anyone at all. Historical information gained from an empathetic, non-judgmental exploration of this topic can be critical to the overall treatment. The following case illustrates how a dual diagnosis – in this instance, depression and an anxiety disorder with opiate/alcohol dependence – and a traumatic personal history can be layered in a complicated pattern:

A 32-year-old woman was admitted to the inpatient psychiatric unit with depression and anxiety, in the context of a substantial history of alcohol and opiate use. Alcohol use had been rampant in her family, and she had vowed to herself that she would avoid the problems she had seen in her parents. In recent years, though, she had succumbed to heavy opiate use after opiates were prescribed for headaches. She had also recently witnessed the death of her brother in a fire, and developed post-traumatic stress disorder (PTSD) symptoms in the aftermath of that tragedy. This in turn led her to begin drinking heavily on top of the opiates. She became aware of a strong craving for alcohol and, out of shame, began to hide her use from her immediate family. She described herself as "amazed" at how all of this had developed, given her resolve to "be different" from her parents. Once the patient was hospitalized and detoxified from alcohol and opiates, she confided a long history of physical and emotional abuse at the hands of her alcoholic parents. The trauma of her brother's death had reawakened many of the memories and feelings associated with the childhood abuse. Now that she was "clean," discussions with her on the unit about her brother's death led to deep catharsis and relief. It was clear that her normal grief response had been delayed by substance use and the associated limbic numbing. An antidepressant was started for both the PTSD and depressive symptoms, and quetiapine was used for sedation at bedtime when her flashbacks were at their worst. But perhaps most important was the support she received in the groups on the unit. She composed a letter to her deceased brother that she read to the group members who responded with empathy and validation of her feelings.

Assessing for PTSD symptoms in patients with long-standing addictions will give a fairly high yield [25–27]. Alertness is also warranted for social phobia symptoms in a patient with a SUD [28]. A phobic patient may self-medicate with substances to quell social anxiety, the same anxiety that may now re-emerge and interfere with the patient's ability to connect with therapy groups on the inpatient unit and to participate in recovery groups after discharge from the hospital.

Patients admitted with symptoms suggesting use of illicit substances or alcohol should be screened for the presence of Axis II traits/disorders, which strongly associate with SUDs [29]. Borderline personality disorder (BPD) in particular has an increased risk of co-morbid SUD [30]. Early detection of a BPD diagnosis is recommended as patients with BPD and co-morbid addiction can provide some of the most difficult treatment challenges on the inpatient unit [31]. In order to prevent the patient's regression on the unit, the hospitalization for the BPD/SUD patient needs to be highly structured, relatively brief, and focused on motivating the patient towards sobriety/abstinence. Interestingly, BPD traits may decrease considerably on the unit with detoxification and abstinence, sometimes even to the point where criteria for the personality disorder are no longer met. However, there is a substantial sub-set of patients with more engrained borderline features in whom substance use is one of many enduring signs of poor impulse control and ego weakness.

How can motivational interviewing be used with dual-diagnosis inpatients?

Motivational interviewing, developed for use with patients with SUDs, is a technique of moving patients, in a non-authoritarian fashion, toward willingness to change habits and behaviors. As a style of interviewing and counseling, it contrasts with less effective purely confrontational approaches, which often lead to arguments and greater resistance in SUD patients. Motivational interviewing stresses the concepts of empathic listening, reframing, and elicitation of patient ambivalence about drug/alcohol use [32, 33]. Motivational interviewing does not preclude the clinician from presenting his/her accumulated evidence for a SUD to the patient, as long as this is done with the same empathic, non-judgmental stance as the rest of the interview. The basic principles of motivational interviewing are not difficult to master and can be readily adapted for use on an inpatient psychiatric unit. Dual-diagnosis patients with deficits in executive functioning or reality testing from severe psychiatric illness may need added support and extrinsic motivators to accept substance use treatment [34].

How important is medical evaluation of inpatients with dual diagnosis?

Abnormalities on the routine laboratory tests and the urine drug screen – which should be standard with all patients admitted to an inpatient unit – can be the first tip-off to a SUD. Specific labs to examine for excessive alcohol use include mean corpuscular volume (MCV), gamma-glutamyltransferase (GGT), liver transaminases, high density lipoprotein, and percent carbohydrate-deficient transferrin (%CDT) [35]. As a general rule, positive values on several (or all) of these measures is much stronger evidence of an alcohol problem than just one or two of them [36].

The medical evaluation of a patient with SUD is similar to that of the routine psychiatric inpatient, but with heightened attention to physical complications of substance use. Thorough evaluation of the patient's medical status is necessary due to the number of commonly occurring end-organ effects of the major categories of SUDs (Table 7.1). Many of the medical/physical

Table 7.1 Physical complications of substance use disorders [37–42]

Alcohol	Liver damage, increased risk of GI cancers, hypertension, cardiovascular disease (including cardiomyopathy), gastritis, anemia/leucopenia/thrombocytopenia, peripheral neuropathy, myopathy, dementia, cerebellar degeneration, withdrawal syndromes (including delirium tremens, seizures)
Cannabis	Airway and GI tract cancers associated with smoking
Opiates	CNS toxicity leading to cognitive impairment, HIV and infections with IV use, renal disease
Amphetamines and cocaine	Hepatic disease, cardiovascular disease, stroke, seizures, renal disease/failure, hyperpyrexia (potentially fatal), nasal perforations (from snorted cocaine)
Inhalants (includes glue, paints, correction fluid, gasoline, butane)	Cortical/cerebellar damage, nerve damage, renal damage, hepatitis, bone marrow suppression
Sedative/hypnotics	Respiratory depression, coma, seizures
Hallucinogens	Cardiac arrest, renal failure (from rhabdomyolysis with PCP), persistent neurocognitive effects, NMS and/or catatonia (with LSD)
Anabolic/androgenic steroids	Acne, gynecomastia, testicular atrophy

CNS = central nervous system; GI = gastrointestinal; HIV = human immunodeficiency virus; IV = intravenous; LSD = lysergic acid diethylamide; NMS = neuroleptic malignant syndrome; PCP = phencyclidine

complications that accompany alcohol/substance use are serious, and some are potentially lethal. The comprehensive inpatient medical evaluation of the SUD or dual-diagnosis patient should include a detailed review of systems, a physical examination, and laboratory testing. Behaviors associated with SUDS increase the risk for blood-borne infections and sexually transmitted diseases. A thorough evaluation may pick up early symptoms of end-organ damage from alcohol or substances.

What are important considerations in managing patients with alcohol dependence?

Alcohol-related symptoms can be variable, depending upon where the patient is in the spectrum from acute intoxication, through withdrawal, to the abstinence syndrome. A major task in the care of patients with significant alcohol

Table 7.2 Factors that indicate primary psychiatric disorder [44]

Clear history of symptoms that preceded the substance use

Report (from patient or collateral source) of periods of symptoms during periods of abstinence/sobriety

Symptoms are not those typically associated with the particular substance used by patient

Strong family history for the suspected primary psychiatric disorder

Symptoms persist longer than expected after withdrawal/abstinence in the hospital

dependence, with or without the presence of a co-morbid psychiatric disorder, is to watch carefully for withdrawal. The most severe form of withdrawal is delirium tremens, a medical emergency that requires transfer to a monitored bed on a medical unit. To lessen the risk of severe withdrawal or Wernicke's encephalopathy, inpatient psychiatric admitting orders should include frequent vital signs, prophylaxis with a benzodiazepine, folate 1 mg daily, and thiamine 100 mg intramuscularly (IM) for three days followed by 100 mg by mouth daily.

Co-occurrence of alcohol dependence with severe mental disorders is common. Patients with bipolar disorder and schizophrenia carry a lifetime risk of developing alcohol dependence of 28% and 26% respectively [5]. The treatment of a known major psychiatric disorder need not be delayed on the inpatient unit because of co-occurrence with alcohol dependence. Concurrent aggressive treatment of mania or psychotic states is often necessary even while treatment for alcohol withdrawal is initiated.

On the other hand, management of depressive symptoms in the context of alcohol withdrawal is not straightforward. Acutely intoxicated patients can look quite despondent, and as mentioned are at elevated risk for suicide, because of the depressant effect of alcohol itself. This state may clear within a week without the need for an antidepressant. The clinician can be guided by looking at the factors that increase the probability that the patient has a depression that is independent of the SUD (Table 7.2). For example, a patient may have a strong family history of mood disorders, may continue to show vegetative symptoms of depression following inpatient detoxification, and/or may report past periods of depression during times of abstinence. An antidepressant should not be withheld from such a patient during the inpatient psychiatric stay.

There also will be a substantial group of patients in whom chronic drinking has led to turmoil in various arenas of their life: work, legal, and family. They are at risk for adjustment disorders and will require the activation of mental health services and other social supports. In response to the therapeutic milieu and groups and activities on the psychiatric unit, these patients often exhibit a brightening of mood. Although this improvement may be punctuated with brief depressive regressions in the face of the stresses they face while on the unit, such as a "bad" phone call, this group of patients will exhibit a gradually more sustained positive mood that does not require antidepressant treatment.

Disulfiram, acamprosate, and naltrexone are three agents that have been approved for use in alcohol dependence. These medications are only infrequently initiated on the inpatient psychiatric unit, but perhaps should be considered more often. Detailed review of these medications, and of other various pharmacologic agents that have been used to promote sobriety, is beyond the scope of this book and is available elsewhere [43].

What about benzodiazepine use/dependence?

Patients who abuse benzodiazepines may have defects in their ability to process and tolerate emotions [45]. They may present as drug-seeking in their behavior on the unit and as "high maintenance" in their dealings with nursing staff. A primary issue for sedative-addicted patients is that they almost literally do not know what their own feelings are or how to deal with unpleasant affective states that arise with abstinence.

Pharmacologic management of benzodiazepine addiction and associated anxiety and withdrawal symptoms may involve the use of initial equivalent doses of a short-acting benzodiazepine, with predictable metabolism, such as lorazepam. Some substance abuse centers are now utilizing phenobarbital, which is less reinforcing than benzodiazepines, as an alternative to lorazepam for acute withdrawal – provided the patient has intact hepatic and pulmonary functioning [46]. Off-label use of quetiapine in doses of 25 to 50 mg three to four times daily can be helpful with underlying anxiety, but will do little for withdrawal symptoms. Similarly, beta-blockers such as atenolol or propranolol are primarily useful for peripheral manifestations of anxiety, not necessarily the anxiety itself. Gabapentin, in off-label use, also has mild prophylactic action against anxiety symptoms.

Many benzodiazepine-dependent patients will have an underlying anxiety disorder. In these instances of dual diagnosis it is especially important to be versed in the use of these non-benzodiazepine medications (Table 7.3). Patients are often cognitively impaired from their long-term addiction and will need to hear repeatedly that their recovery will be a protracted process, taking weeks to months.

Patients with dual diagnosis of a SUD and schizophrenia or bipolar disorder are also prone to develop addiction to prescribed benzodiazepines [19]. Consequently, for this group of patients, inpatient psychiatrists should be wary of initiating benzodiazepines and should entertain alternative classes of medications or non-pharmacologic treatments for anxiety symptoms.

Table 7.3 Alternatives to benzodiazepines for anxiety [47–52]

Medication	Comments
Antihistamines (e.g., diphenhydramine)	can help with sleep
	anticholinergic side effects limit use
Atypical antipsychotics	off-label use
	some experts question exposing patients without psychosis to metabolic or motor side effects
Buspirone	patients previously on benzodiazepines may not respond well
	takes a few weeks for effect
SSRIs and SNRIs	useful for generalized anxiety and panic symptoms
	take several weeks for effect
	possible weight gain and sexual side effects
Mirtazapine	good for sedation and sleep
	weight gain and over-sedation can limit use
Tricyclic antidepressants	take several weeks for effect
	side effects limit use for some
	lethal in overdose
Gabapentin	off-label use
	useful for anxiety and sedation
	relatively weight neutral
Pregabalin	off-label use
	industry-sponsored studies show comparable to SNRIs
	may work within a week
	expensive if not covered by insurance

How does one manage opiate dependence in psychiatric inpatients?

Co-morbid opiate use disorders occur commonly in major psychiatric ill-nesses and obscure the overall clinical presentation. For this reason, addic-tion to opiates, prescribed or bought on the street, should be included in the check-list of reasons why a given patient with a major psychiatric illness has failed to respond to adequate pharmacologic treatment. A patient admitted to an inpatient unit with treatment-resistant depression or refractory psychosis may therefore need to be detoxified from opiate medications. Nowadays the state-of-the-art treatment entails use of buprenorphine, an opiate agent with high affinity for the μ-opioid receptor and lower abuse potential than other opioids [53]. Because the co-occurrence of opiate abuse and psychiatric syndromes is so prevalent, many psychiatrists have familiarized themselves with the use of buprenorphine through training seminars and courses.

Awareness of the role of co-morbidities has led some psychiatrists to focus on a particularly difficult group of patients: those with "triple diagnosis," the co-occurrence of substance use, depression, and chronic pain. Buprenorphine may have a special function in the treatment of these complex patients; a four-times-per-day dosing of buprenorphine can often simultaneously address chronic pain and narcotic cravings [54].

Can cocaine or amphetamine users be admitted to an inpatient psychiatric unit?

Patients who abuse these stimulant drugs will present to the hospital in one of two states: intoxicated or in withdrawal (the so-called "crash") [55, 56]. In the intoxicated state, patients may appear hypomanic and paranoid, and show autonomic signs of activation. In the abstinence state, patients will have been depleted of catecholamines and will want to sleep all day and night, sometimes for the first several days on the unit. Also contributing to this state is the fact that they have been running full blast for days on end and are sleep deprived. This withdrawal syndrome does not usually require specific medical intervention. Long-term use of cocaine or amphetamine can lead to paranoia/ psychosis and affective states that are very difficult to distinguish from a primary mood or psychotic disorder, and patients may require months of abstinence for resolution of the symptoms. Amphetamine and cocaine SUDs can co-exist with primary psychiatric disorders as well. Bipolar disorder patients may gravitate to cocaine and amphetamines in an attempt to simulate their manic states, or conversely, to self-medicate their depressions [57]. When patients with bona fide schizophrenia are abusing these drugs on top of their underlying illness, it may render their psychotic symptoms treatment resistant [58].

The college age group is particularly prone to abuse of prescription stimulants for attention-deficit/hyperactivity disorder (ADHD), which may be sold or distributed by students in the dormitories [59]. The long-acting preparations of the various stimulant medications are less rewarding/reinforcing and less likely to be "diverted" to non-patients than pure dextroamphetamine or methylphenidate. Patients may claim they have untreated ADHD because they experience improved concentration with use of cocaine or amphetamines, and may use this personal "self-medication" theory to justify their substance use. Despite whatever positive effects stimulant abuse is bringing them, a definitive diagnosis of ADHD will require further evaluation after a period of abstinence from the "treatment." Patients who are assessed to have stimulant abuse *and* ADHD can be offered second-line alternatives to stimulants, such as atomoxetine or bupropion [60].

What about cannabis use in psychiatric inpatients?

Cannabis is a commonly used substance in psychiatric inpatients, and often as part of a polysubstance use pattern. The age of first use of cannabis has been decreasing in recent years, with nicotine serving as the gateway for use in adolescents. Cannabis use in isolation seldom leads to an inpatient psychiatric admission; treatment for primary cannabis dependence takes place in outpatient substance clinics. However, it is important to recognize cannabis use as part of a dual-diagnosis pattern in inpatients with mood disorders and psychotic disorders. In both groups, cannabis use can lead to a more refractory presentation and can prolong the hospital stay [61–63]. Cannabis use has also been associated with an earlier onset of prodromal symptoms and psychotic symptoms in schizophrenia [64]. Cannabis may also be a causative agent for gray matter loss and cognitive decline in patients with schizophrenia, consequences of cannabis use that should be communicated to patients and their families [65].

What are signs and symptoms of anabolic-androgenic steroid use?

Young male athletes, bodybuilders in particular, may use anabolic-androgenic steroids (AAS) to enhance body mass and muscularity. Regular use leads to mood instability with hypomanic and depressive phases that correspond to "cycles" of use followed by withdrawal from the drug. Accordingly, AAS use should be considered in the differential diagnosis of bipolar disorder. Patients using AAS may present to the emergency department in states of intense irritability or violent behavior, so-called "roid rage." Characteristics on the physical examination of patients using AAS include improbable degrees of fat-free muscularity, acne, gynecomastia, and testicular atrophy (which is associated with sterility and impotence) [42]. Patients with AAS addiction may suffer from body-image distortions, and in that respect are thought to resemble women with eating disorders and/or patients with body dysmorphic disorder [66] (Table 7.4.).

Table 7.4 *In our experience...* Hints for treating dual-diagnosis inpatients

Be prepared to deal with denial of substance use by patients. Some of our patients who are positive for cocaine try to convince us that it was "the only time in my life I ever used" or that "someone must have laced my cigarettes."

Address both the primary psychiatric illness as well as the substance use. Treatment will fail if you deal exclusively with one or the other.

Use family for collateral history... though some patients with addictions have burned all their bridges with family and friends.

Direct patients to use support groups after discharge. Regular attendance at Alcoholics Anonymous can help patients tremendously.

Become adept at using non-addictive agents and non-pharmacologic treatments for various psychiatric symptoms in dual-diagnosis patients.

Remember: Substance use is *common*. Have a high index of suspicion for SUD in inpatients when puzzled by the history, presentation, or (lack of) response to treatment.

References

1. Lehman A, Myers C, Corty E & Thompson J. Prevalence and patterns of "dual diagnosis" among psychiatric inpatients. *Comprehensive Psychiatry*, **35**:2 (1994), 106–12.

2. Kelly J & Westerhoff C. Does it matter how we refer to individuals with substance-related conditions? A randomized study of two commonly used terms. *International Journal of Drug Policy*, **21**:3 (2010), 202–7.

3. Bulkley L D. Syphilis occurring in connection with other diseases of the skin. In: Medical Society of the State of New York, ed., *Transactions of the Medical Society of the State of New York*. Syracuse, NY: The Syracuse Journal Company; 1887.

4. Kessler R. The epidemiology of dual diagnosis. *Biological Psychiatry*, **56**:10 (2004), 730–7.

5. Buckley P & Brown E. Prevalence and consequences of dual diagnosis. *Journal of Clinical Psychiatry*, **67**:7 (2006), e01.

6. Breslow R E, Klinger B I & Erickson B J. Acute intoxication and substance abuse among patients presenting to a psychiatric emergency service. *General Hospital Psychiatry*, **18**:3 (1996), 183–91.

7. Budney A, Hughes J, Moore B & Vandrey R. Review of the validity and significance of cannabis withdrawal syndrome. *American Journal of Psychiatry*, **161**:11 (2004), 1967.

8. McKeon A, Frye M & Delanty N. The alcohol withdrawal syndrome. *British Medical Journal*, **79**:8 (2008), 854.

9. Wright S, Gournay K, Glorney E & Thornicroft G. Dual diagnosis in the suburbs: prevalence, need, and in-patient service use. *Social Psychiatry and Psychiatric Epidemiology*, **35**:7 (2000), 297–304.

10. Mordal J, Bramness J, Holm B & Mørland J. Drugs of abuse among acute psychiatric and medical admissions: laboratory based identification of prevalence and drug influence. *General Hospital Psychiatry*, **30**:1 (2008), 55–60.

11. Caton C L, Drake R E, Hasin D S *et al*. Differences between early-phase primary psychotic disorders with concurrent substance use and substance-induced psychoses. *Archives of General Psychiatry*, **62**:2 (2005), 137–45.

12. Caton C L, Hasin D S, Shrout P E *et al*. Stability of early-phase primary psychotic disorders with concurrent substance use and substance-induced psychosis. *British Journal of Psychiatry*, **190** (2007), 105–11.

13. Renner J A. How to train residents to identify and treat dual diagnosis patients. *Biological Psychiatry*, **56**:10 (2004), 810–16.

14. Ziedonis D. Integrated treatment of co-occurring mental illness and addiction: clinical intervention, program, and system perspectives. *CNS Spectrums*, **9**:12 (2004), 892–904, 925.

15. Cornelius J, Clark D, Salloum I, Bukstein O & Kelly T. Management of suicidal behavior in alcoholism. *Clinical Neuroscience Research*, **1**:5 (2001), 381–6.

16. Goldberg J F, Singer T M & Garno J L. Suicidality and substance abuse in affective disorders. *Journal of Clinical Psychiatry*, **62**:Suppl. 25 (2001), 35–43.

17. Duffy J & Kreitman N. Risk factors for suicide and undetermined death among in-patient alcoholics in Scotland. *Addiction*, **88**:6 (1993), 757–66.

18. Schneider B. Substance use disorders and risk for completed suicide. *Archives of Suicide Research*, **13**:4 (2009), 303–16.

19. Brunette M F, Noordsy D L, Xie H & Drake R E. Benzodiazepine use and abuse among patients with severe mental illness and co-occurring substance use disorders. *Psychiatric Services*, **54**:10 (2003), 1395–401.

20. Hallahan B, Murray I & McDonald C. Benzodiazepine and hypnotic prescribing in an acute adult psychiatric in-patient unit. *Psychiatric Bulletin*, **33**:1 (2009), 12.

21. Drake R, Mercer-McFadden C, Mueser K, McHugo G & Bond G. Review of integrated mental health and substance abuse treatment for patients with dual disorders. *Schizophrenia Bulletin*, **24** (1998), 589–608.

22. Osher F & Drake R. Reversing a history of unmet needs: approaches to care for persons with co-occurring addictive and mental disorders. *American Journal of Orthopsychiatry*, **66**:1 (1996), 4–11.

23. Renner J A Jr, Karam-Hage M, Levinson M, Craig T & Eld B. What do psychiatric residents think of addiction psychiatry as a career? *Academic Psychiatry*, **33**:2 (2009), 139–42.

24. Tinsley J A. Workforce information on addiction psychiatry graduates. *Academic Psychiatry*, **28**:1 (2004), 56–9.

25. Brown P, Recupero P & Stout R. PTSD substance abuse comorbidity and treatment utilization. *Addictive Behaviors*, **20**:2 (1995), 251–4.

26. Najavits L, Weiss R & Shaw S. The link between substance abuse and posttraumatic stress disorder in women. A research review. *American Journal on Addictions*, **6**:4 (1997), 273–83.

27. Kofoed L, Friedman M J & Peck R. Alcoholism and drug abuse in patients with PTSD. *Psychiatric Quarterly*, **64**:2 (1993), 151–71.

28. Kessler R C, McGonagle K A, Zhao S *et al.* Lifetime and 12-month prevalence of DSM-III-R psychiatric disorders in the United States. Results from the National Comorbidity Survey. *Archive of General Psychiatry*, **51**:1 (1994), 8–19.

29. Regier D A, Farmer M E, Rae D S *et al.* Comorbidity of mental disorders with alcohol and other drug abuse. Results from the Epidemiologic Catchment Area (ECA) Study. *Journal of the American Medical Association*, **264**:19 (1990), 2511–18.

30. Grilo C, Martino S, Walker M *et al.* Controlled study of psychiatric comorbidity in psychiatrically hospitalized young adults with substance use disorders. *American Journal of Psychiatry*, **154**:9 (1997), 1305.

31. Zanarini M C, Frankenburg F R, Hennen J, Reich D B & Silk K R. Axis I comorbidity in patients with borderline personality disorder: 6-year follow-up and prediction of time to remission. *American Journal of Psychiatry*, **161**:11 (2004), 2108–14.

32. Miller W R. Motivational interviewing: research, practice, and puzzles. *Addictive Behaviors*, **21**:6 (1996), 835–42.

33. Rubak S, Sandbæk A, Lauritzen T & Christensen B. Motivational interviewing: a systematic review and meta-analysis. *British Journal of General Practice*, **55**:513 (2005), 305.

34. DiClemente C, Nidecker M & Bellack A. Motivation and the stages of change among individuals with severe mental illness and substance abuse disorders. *Journal of Substance Abuse Treatment*, **34**:1 (2008), 25–35.

35. Allen J P & Litten R Z. The role of laboratory tests in alcoholism treatment. *Journal of Substance Abuse Treatment*, **20**:1 (2001), 81–5.

36. Spiegel D, Dhadwal N & Gill F. "I'm sober, Doctor, really": Best biomarkers for underreported alcohol use. *Current Psychiatry*, **7**:9 (2008), 15.

37. Akmal M, Valdin J R, McCarron M M & Massry S G. Rhabdomyolysis with and without acute renal failure in patients with phencyclidine intoxication. *American Journal of Nephrology*, **1**:2 (1981), 91–6.

38. Baigent M F. Physical complications of substance abuse: what the psychiatrist needs to know. *Current Opinion in Psychiatry*, **16**:3 (2003), 291–6.

39. Behan W M, Bakheit A M, Behan P O & More I A. The muscle findings in the neuroleptic malignant syndrome associated with lysergic acid diethylamide. *Journal of Neurology, Neurosurgery & Psychiatry*, **54**:8 (1991), 741–3.

40. Devlin R J & Henry J A. Clinical review: major consequences of illicit drug consumption. *Critical Care*, **12**:1 (2008), 202.

41. Lieber C S. Medical disorders of alcoholism. *England Journal of Medicine*, **333**:16 (1995), 1058–65.

42. Pope H & Kanayama G. Bodybuilding's dark side: clues to anabolic steroid use. *Current Psychiatry*, **3**:12 (2004), 12–20.

43. Heilig M & Egli M. Pharmacological treatment of alcohol dependence: target symptoms and target mechanisms. *Pharmacology and Therapeutics*, **111**:3 (2006), 855–76.

44. Weiss R. Identifying and diagnosing co-occurring disorders. *CNS Spectrums*, **13**:4 Suppl 6 (2008), 4–6.

45. Khantzian E J. The self-medication hypothesis of substance use disorders: a reconsideration and recent applications. *Harvard Review of Psychiatry*, **4**:5 (1997), 231–44.

46. Rodgers J E & Crouch M A. Phenobarbital for alcohol withdrawal syndrome. *American Journal of Health-System Pharmacy*, **56**:2 (1999), 175–8.

47. Sajatovic M. Treatment for mood and anxiety disorders: quetiapine and aripiprazole. *Current Psychiatry Reports*, **5**:4 (2003), 320–6.

48. Gao K, Muzina D, Gajwani P & Calabrese J. Efficacy of typical and atypical antipsychotics for primary and co-morbid anxiety symptoms or disorders: a review. *Journal of Clinical Psychiatry*, **67**:9 (2006), 1327–40.

49. Hoffman E & Mathew S. Anxiety disorders: a comprehensive review of pharmacotherapies. *Mount Sinai Journal of Medicine*, **75**:3 (2008), 248–62.

50. Addolorato G, Caputo F, Capristo E *et al.* Baclofen efficacy in reducing alcohol craving and intake: a preliminary double-blind randomized controlled study. *Alcohol and Alcoholism*, **37**:5 (2002), 504.

51. Flannery B, Garbutt J, Cody M *et al.* Baclofen for alcohol dependence: a preliminary open-label study. Alcoholism, *Clinical and Experimental Research*, **28**:10 (2004), 1517–23.

52. Strawn J & Geracioti T Jr. The treatment of generalized anxiety disorder with pregabalin, an atypical anxiolytic. *Neuropsychiatric Disease and Treatment*, **3**:2 (2007), 237.

53. George S & Day E. Buprenorphine in the treatment of opioid dependence. *British Journal of Hospital Medicine*, **68**:11 (2007), 594–7.

54. Malinoff H L, Barkin R L & Wilson G. Sublingual buprenorphine is effective in the treatment of chronic pain syndrome. *American Journal of Therapeutics*, **12**:5 (2005), 379–84.

55. Gray S, Fatovich D, McCoubrie D & Daly F. Amphetamine-related presentations to an inner-city tertiary emergency department: a prospective evaluation. *Medical Journal of Australia*, **186**:7 (2007), 336.

56. McGregor C, Srisurapanont M, Jittiwutikarn J *et al.* The nature, time course and severity of methamphetamine withdrawal. *Addiction*, **100**:9 (2005), 1320.

57. Brown E, Nejtek V, Perantie D & Bobadilla L. Quetiapine in bipolar disorder and cocaine dependence. *Bipolar Disorders*, **4**:6 (2002), 406–11.

58. Elkis H. Treatment-resistant schizophrenia. *Psychiatric Clinics of North America*, **30**:3 (2007), 511–33.

59. McCabe S, Knight J, Teter C & Wechsler H. Non-medical use of prescription stimulants among US college students: prevalence and correlates from a national survey. *Addiction*, **100**:1 (2005), 96–106.

60. Wilens T E. Impact of ADHD and its treatment on substance abuse in adults. *Journal of Clinical Psychiatry*, **65**:3 (2004), 38–45.

61. Raphael B, Wooding S, Stevens G & Connor J. Comorbidity: cannabis and complexity. *Journal of Psychiatric Practice*, **11**:3 (2005), 161–76.

62. Winklbaur B, Ebner N, Sachs G, Thau K & Fischer G. Substance abuse in patients with schizophrenia. *Dialogues in Clinical Neuroscience*, **8**:1 (2006), 37–43.

63. Di Forti M, Morrison P D, Butt A & Murray R M. Cannabis use and psychiatric and cognitive disorders: the chicken or the egg? *Current Opinion in Psychiatry*, **20**:3 (2007), 228–34.

64. Compton M T, Kelley M E, Ramsay C E *et al.* Association of pre-onset cannabis, alcohol, and tobacco use with age at onset of prodrome and age at onset of psychosis in first-episode patients. *American Journal of Psychiatry*, **166**:11 (2009), 1251–7.

65. Freedman R. Cannabis, inhibitory neurons, and the progressive course of schizophrenia. *American Journal of Psychiatry*, **165**:4 (2008), 416–19.

66. Pope H G Jr, Gruber A J, Choi P, Olivardia R & Phillips K A. Muscle dysmorphia. An underrecognized form of body dysmorphic disorder. *Psychosomatics*, **38**:6 (1997), 548–57.

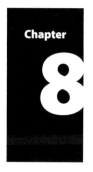

Chapter

8

The young adult on the inpatient unit

When specific diagnoses are mentioned, we are referring to diagnoses and criteria as listed in the *Diagnostic and Statistical Manual of Mental Disorders*, 4th edition, text revision (DSM-IV-TR) unless otherwise specified.

How should the term "young adult" be defined?

In the psychiatric literature, "young adults" are often defined by age alone, generally between 18 and 25 years of age. However, a more fluid conception would allow for individual variations in rates of emotional/cognitive development, and would factor in the influence of societal and cultural forces that may delay independent adult functioning [1]. The heterogeneity of young adulthood is not hard to see; most clinicians have encountered 17-year-olds who act and think like they are 21, and vice versa. From the legal standpoint, in most Western cultures, 18 is the age of majority, at which point entrance into contractual agreements is allowed and adult responsibility for criminal behavior is demanded. Yet, brain maturation continues at least into the early 20s [2, 3], including ongoing myelination, dendritic arborization and pruning that lead to increased executive functioning and greater frontal lobe control over limbic emotional centers [4]. Thus, many young adult patients do not yet have a fully functioning "adult brain."

Young adults who have progressed through late adolescence without major developmental interferences enter a stage in which they begin to see the world through the eyes of a grown up. They are expected to have mastered emotional separation from their family to the point where parents no longer exert undue influence on their judgment and decision-making. By this stage, moral standards, religious/philosophical attitudes, and a burgeoning worldview are in place and are not contingent upon or sustained by the family's endorsement [1]. Young adults who are on track developmentally have also progressed beyond Erikson's adolescent stage of identity formation and are establishing intimacy, including patterns of fulfillment of sexual needs [5].

Table 8.1 Tasks of young adulthood

Consolidation of core identity (including sexual identity)

Continued emotional separation from parents and reassessment of family values/ideologies

Achievement of a dyadic love relationship

Satisfactory early parenthood (if chosen)

Establishment of vocation/career or advanced schooling/training in chosen area

Stable executive functioning including impulse control, affect regulation

While the precise timing of the transition from late adolescence to young adulthood varies from person to person, on the whole this is a shift marked externally by a relatively secure foothold in adult roles and responsibilities, such as education/career, a dyadic partnership, parenthood, and contribution to one's community (Table 8.1). Internally, young adulthood is represented by increased stability and consolidation of the post-adolescent developmental accomplishments outlined by Erikson and others, including those in the areas of relatedness and identity formation. Compared to late adolescents, young adults show a greater ability to tolerate strong affects or need states without resorting to regressive behaviors. In addition, with passage into adulthood, young people are forging their own paths, and are increasingly independent of parental influence and constraints.

Not only is there considerable variation in functioning *among* young adult inpatients, but clinicians will also observe inconsistencies *within* an individual patient in terms of functioning in different domains of adult coping and thinking. For instance, a young adult patient with obsessive–compulsive traits may have a highly developed moral sense but impaired flexibility in dealing with new situations. Or, although a given patient may have developed mature "contextualized" moral reasoning, this capacity can be lost with the stress of an acute psychiatric illness. One also sees variability in young adult patients' reactions to being hospitalized, with some patients seeming to luxuriate in the dependent regression and secondary gain for illness, while others hate the patient role and push for a premature discharge from the hospital.

Can the age of "young adulthood" be delayed or quickened by external factors?

Some scholars contend that college prolongs adolescence, or that adoption of adult responsibilities, such as work or marriage, hastens the onset of adulthood. They argue that for young persons in industrialized countries, "young adulthood" should be called "emerging adulthood" to account for the delays in embarking on true adult responsibilities during a period of exploration, schooling, and continued reliance on parental support [1]. However, while societal factors appear to have some effect on maturation rates, the physiologically based unfolding of mature brain functioning is a more powerful influence on the progression toward adult functioning. An 18-year-old may have adult responsibilities but still be awaiting the fundamental brain development associated with adult coping skills and capacity for mature appraisal. Someone who is married and working at age 18 is performing adult tasks, but is likely functioning as an adolescent in many respects. In addition, there are 21-year-old college students who run the university newspaper, organize various clubs and activities, or complete publishable research projects, and who may be functioning at a more adult level than some of their same-age peers who got married and entered the workforce right after high school.

What are the special problems associated with the psychiatric hospitalization of a young adult?

Young adult inpatients may be deemed competent from a legal standpoint, but may not be making adult-level decisions. Some young adult patients with immature judgment capacity are unable to rationally discuss their treatment plan with the inpatient team. One of the major developmental tasks of late adolescence and young adulthood is a transformation in the perception of parental figures, which allows figures in authority to be viewed as helpful and wise but not "controlling." Young adult patients may still be struggling with resolving this ambivalence toward authority figures, and as a consequence may seem to be fighting against the treatment recommendations. Challenging clinical scenarios occur when such a patient is making impulse-driven decisions but is unwilling to allow family involvement, and pushes for a premature discharge from the hospital against medical advice.

Hospitalized young adults also frequently do not have adequate social supports. Many young adults are in a fluid state in which they have rightfully achieved some separation from their family of origin, but have not established a new nuclear family of their own. Reticent about discussing their illness openly, they are reluctant to turn toward friends to fill in the gap. On the most severe end of the spectrum are those young adults with chronic psychiatric illnesses, who are often estranged from their families and socially isolated from their peers. With either of these circumstances, both the psychiatrist and the inpatient unit social worker may find it difficult to access and assess a support network for collateral history and discharge planning.

Many young adults will have difficulty embracing the idea of a psychiatric hospitalization. With some justification, they might view the hospital as a place that robs them of their hard-won independence in judgment and decision-making. Also being in the hospital quite literally restricts their freedom and mobility. Moreover, most acute care inpatient psychiatric units have prudently restricted sexual interactions on the unit, due to medical–legal and clinical concerns, including the risks of sexually transmitted diseases and pregnancy, and the potential for exploitative relationships [6]. Such policies are particularly difficult for testosterone-driven young males who are now in close quarters with a multitude of young female social workers, female medical and nursing students – and, of course, female patients. Young adult males are not alone in struggling with sexual frustration; young adult females, especially those prone toward acting out, may have similar frustrations with hospital rules.

Female young adult inpatients in particular may react negatively to any threat to their independence [7], and experience hospitalization as undercutting their self-esteem. Young women are actively involved in separating psychologically from their mothers (in particular), and may be sensitive to perceived intrusions by female staff. Taking these developmental needs into account, the best approach toward young adult females on the unit is one of active listening and collaborative engagement rather than an overly directive manner.

Awareness that we, as humans, are interconnected with others may be lacking in the young adult patient. As adolescents enter adult life, they often have a sense of self-sufficiency and the illusion that they do not need external input to get help with problems. This deficit in mature sensibility is also related to the unresolved conflict in the arena of autonomy versus independence, which can lead to a perception of the hospitalization as a clamping down on the ability to think and function independently. Young adult patients who focus exclusively on the restrictions inherent in a hospitalization will view the inpatient stay as a developmental disruption, and will fail to appreciate the opportunity for personal change and growth when illness is treated. Young adult patients can be counseled that the sacrifices of a hospitalization are ultimately in the service of furthering them along their developmental path by decreasing interference from psychiatric illness. With the development of the therapeutic alliance, most patients will begin to improve their view of hospitalization. With empathetic handling during the inpatient period, young adult patients may ultimately look back on the hospitalization as an unpleasant but necessary interlude that was in their interest (Table 8.2). With certain patients, this insight will only be attained with the quieting, usually with medication treatment, of a severe psychopathologic process such as psychosis, severe depression, or mania.

How do Blos, Erikson, and Winnicott relate to the hospitalization of a young adult?

Peter Blos's classic *On Adolescence* [8] and *The Adolescent Passage* [9] have much to say about the journey through adolescence and the transition to young adulthood. Blos termed this phase "the second individuation," referring

Table 8.2 *In our experience...* Hints for connecting with the young adult patient

Do not talk down to young adults. Instead, communicate that you respect their ideas.

You can always adjust to a more directive stance if the patient shows they are not functioning at an adult level. Patients with severe illness need this, at least temporarily.

Try to avoid medications that can cause weight gain, sexual interference, and/or cognitive slowing.

Help the patient figure out what they want to communicate to their job, college, friends, and family.

Communicate to the patient that you understand that being in the hospital is difficult for busy young adults. Get the patient to outpatient treatment as quickly as possible.

If substance or alcohol use is an issue, avoid being judgmental. Use motivational interviewing techniques.

Remember: Being in the hospital can undermine the young adult's need to be independent. Demonstrate to the patient that you appreciate this.

to its earlier counterpart in the physical separation from the early parental figures, in particular the mother, which occurs in infancy and toddlerhood. He notes that the earlier developmental task has to do with relinquishing the physical presence of the caregiver through motor ability, hunger to learn about the world at large, and a growing capacity to "self-soothe." By way of contrast, Blos states that the transition to young adulthood includes freeing oneself from the "internalized parent" as a governor of thinking and behavior, replacing this image with a renegotiated view of the parents that allows for greater independence. The "third individuation" of young adulthood has been described as further redefinition of self and others through relationships outside the family and education/work [10].

Blos's ideas permeate even our current understanding of adolescent psychology, and can inform our understanding of young adults' reactions to psychiatric illness and hospitalization. When patients suffer from major psychiatric illness requiring hospitalization, staff often see regressive behaviors and attitudes that accompany the loss of capacity to function autonomously. Patients in such a state might see the parents and other authorities as larger-than-life figures that are to be yielded to entirely. Then there is a repeat of the transition from dependent child to independent adult, in which patients, via reaction formation, summarily dismiss these same authority figures. Young adult patients may fluctuate between these two extremes, sometimes acting clingy and needy, while at other times rejecting help from unit staff.

Erik Erikson took the ideas of psychosexual development and ego functioning put forth by Anna Freud and others, and extended them to the sociocultural sphere. This is embodied in his "eight stages of man" [5]. In Eriksonian terms, young adults without significant psychopathology will have successfully traversed the stage of "identity vs. identity diffusion," are completing the tasks of "intimacy vs. isolation," and are beginning to look toward the stage of "generativity vs. stagnation." But serious psychiatric illness will interfere with the young adult's capacity to form and sustain relationships, including the friendships and intimate romantic bonds that are so crucial to this age group. And the self-absorption that accompanies depression certainly makes it difficult to focus on the care and nurturing of the next generation that should mark the transition to Erikson's stage of generativity.

D. W. Winnicott [11] has contributed several concepts that are relevant to inpatient treatment and to the young adult inpatient in particular. His kōan-like aphorism "there is no such thing as a baby," articulates the symbiosis that occurs between mother and infant. This concept of motherhood adds tremendous richness to our understanding of the period of pregnancy and birth in the young adult women who may present to the psychiatric unit. It reminds us that mothers with post-partum depression will have an aspect of their presentation that relates to the trauma of separation from their infants. Even in those with psychiatric illnesses other than depression, distance from their babies may result in an extra layer of separation anxiety and depression. Therefore, psychiatric inpatient units will have to accommodate the need of mothers to remain attached in some fashion to their young infants, either utilizing infant "live-in" programs or liberal visiting hours [12]. Of course, preservation of the mother–baby attachment during the hospitalization has to be balanced with the need of some severely ill young mothers to have a period of time in which they are freed from caregiving responsibilities.

Winnicott describes the mother's contribution to the dyad of mother–child as a "holding environment" that buffers the emotional life of the child and allows strong affects to be tolerated [11]. Certain patients experience the refuge and support of a hospitalization as an analogue to the care they may or may not have received in their early life. In fact, many patients struggle with feelings of abandonment when the time comes for discharge from the hospital. But the hospital can not, and should not, be the "all giving" mother. Winnicott also uses the term "good-enough mothering" to refer to the less than perfect parental attunement that disappoints while still being adequate to foster emotional maturation. The "good-enough hospital" then could be seen as one that satisfies some, but not all, of a patient's needs. It can provide a temporary respite, or "holding environment," from the stressors that led to illness and a safe atmosphere where the patient can heal [13].

Winnicott's most recognized concept is perhaps that of the "transitional object," which refers to the teddy bears and blankets that toddlers carry to ease their transition from the close dyadic relationship with the mother to a relationship with the world at large [14]. Both the transitional object itself and the manner in which it is treated share characteristics with the mother and the child's relationship with the mother. For example, the material from which it is constructed usually is soft and provides for a soothing sensation when held against the face. And, just as the infantile physical tie to the mother is difficult to relinquish, the tattered "blankie" is difficult to discard – though that is its ultimate fate. Some clinicians see a diagnostic marker in the fondness of adult woman patients with borderline personality disorder for the stuffed animals they bring to the hospital, an association that has actually been borne out in a study of the persistence of transitional objects into adult life [15]. However, caution is advised in being too facile with this interpretation in the young adult female patient, who may be using transitional items to deal with the separation processes of young adulthood or to cope with the stress of a hospitalization, and who may not ultimately meet criteria for an Axis II disorder.

What special considerations for young adulthood apply for common psychiatric diagnoses?

Large epidemiologic studies have shown that by young adulthood most major psychiatric illnesses will have made their appearance, with 75% of all adult psychiatric illness beginning in childhood or adolescence [16, 17]. The illnesses described in this volume are the "bread and butter" cases of young adulthood, and the broad rules of treatment described here and elsewhere apply. Nevertheless, there are elements of the diagnosis and treatment of patients from these diagnostic groupings that should be highlighted in the young adult population.

While many young adults with depression on an inpatient unit will have had previous episodes of depressive illness, a first episode of major depression can occur when young adults depart from their home for the first time, like when entering college. Although these patients will likely meet criteria for Major Depressive Disorder, there will invariably be a large contribution from homesickness and difficulty coping on one's own. Many of these patients will not go on to develop a lifetime depressive illness. In the instances in which stress or depression has led to the threat of suicide or total loss of functioning, a brief focused inpatient stay can be used to initiate medication, foster coping skills, and provide psychoeducation about mood disorders. For young adults who are displaying a pattern of recurrent depressions, the hospitalization will also need to focus on acceptance of the chronic nature of the illness and the need for acceptance of the diagnosis and long-term adherence to medications.

Bipolar disorder – mania in particular – is difficult to manage in this age group for a number of reasons. Young adults in a manic state have the physical wherewithal to do serious damage to themselves, others, and property, both prior to admission and on the inpatient unit itself. It is therefore important for staff to be alert to the patient's level of agitation and to be proactive with behavioral interventions and pharmacologic measures from the moment the patient arrives on the unit (see Chapters 1 and 3). One of the hallmarks of bipolar disorder is the denial of illness, a feature that may be particularly prominent in young persons. It is common to see repeated admissions in young adult patients with bipolar disorder due to lack of acceptance of the need for medication and other interventions. Furthermore, onset of bipolar disorder in adolescence appears to be a risk factor for greater impairment in young adulthood [18]. Whether a first episode or a recurrence, the provider's tasks include keeping the treatment regimen simple, addressing the side effects of medication, and building a treatment alliance that allows the clinician to relate to the young adult patient's concerns and to break through the denial of illness.

Borderline personality disorder is expressed most actively in late teenage years and young adulthood, and often leads to the need for inpatient treatment during that period. Perhaps the greatest challenge in treating young adults with borderline personality disorder on the inpatient unit is controlling staff countertransference reactions to the impulsivity, suicidal/self-mutilative behaviors, and inappropriate anger that characterize these patients, especially when they are in crisis [19, 20]. Patients and their families may be reassured to know that the illness is treatable (see Chapter 4) and that many symptoms of the disorder may disappear altogether as patients mature [21]. Clinicians also need to be careful not to mistake the emotional turmoil in normal young people during late adolescence/early adulthood for borderline pathology.

Schizophrenic spectrum illness in young adults presents the patient, the patient's family, and the treating clinician with heart-breaking challenges, including coping with the onset of the illness in these young persons who not only may be unable to return to school or work, but who also may never again reach their previous level of functioning [22]. When treating these first-break patients, clinicians need to be aware of their own feelings of hopelessness so they can help the patient and family deal with what is still seen as a grim diagnosis [23, 24]. First-break patients are at risk for suicidal behaviors as they see their current lives unravel and their future aspirations fade from possibility. (See Chapter 1 for more detailed discussion.) To decrease the probability of a fragile, newly diagnosed schizophrenic patient "falling through the cracks," the patient's transition from the hospital to a day program or outpatient clinic should be as seamless as possible.

Epidemiologic studies have confirmed the clinical observation that young adulthood is a peak onset period for drug and alcohol disorders [25]. Substance use may be part of a young adult pattern of risk taking and sensation seeking that peaks in the early 20s [1]. Many of those so-afflicted find their way to inpatient psychiatric units, where they present with substance-related mood disorders or dual diagnosis disorders. (See Chapter 7.)

A pattern of poor mental health associated with drinking (PMHD) in college students has been described as consisting of a complex of increased alcohol consumption, depression, and stress related to academic performance and health issues [26]. Inpatient psychiatric units need to be sites of recognition of substance and alcohol use in this population. College-aged students have to deal with a campus culture that promotes drinking, which is seen as part of the rite of passage for these young people. Students may perceive it inimical to their college social life *not* to use drugs or alcohol. Many young people can transverse this period in their lives without difficulty, but the small percentage with genetic or other predispositions to addiction will be casualties of this environment. When these patients present to the inpatient unit, their denial of addiction is often prominent. Young persons may respond more readily to a motivational interviewing style [27] (see Chapter 7) that meets the patients "where they are," and allows for a discussion of a patient's perceived pros and cons of substance use, as opposed to the paternalistic medical warnings clinicians are tempted to offer.

What are the special considerations with medications in young adults?

Young adults are likely to be able to tolerate most psychotropic medications in regularly prescribed dosages. Nonetheless, some side effects are more common in the younger age group. Young males, especially those with high muscle mass, show a greater incidence of extra-pyramidal symptoms (EPS) [28]. This is especially true with the traditional antipsychotic medications, but can occur as well with atypicals. In addition, there has been recent attention to the emergence of suicidal thoughts and actions in adolescents and young adults who are beginning antidepressants [29–31]. These patients and their families should be warned of this possibility, and inpatient staff should closely monitor the patient when antidepressants are initiated.

Consideration of risks and benefits of various medications during pregnancy and breast-feeding is commonly necessary when treating young adult females on an inpatient unit. The risks of untreated illness further complicate the equation. Therefore, awareness of these issues is extremely important when treating all young adult women who are or will be sexually active – whether or not they are post-partum and breast-feeding, pregnant, or trying to get pregnant. Pregnancy testing should be part of the routine admission evaluation of all women in this group, and frank discussion about birth control is necessary by the date of discharge. A full treatment of this topic is beyond the scope of this manual, but the authors direct readers' attention to the cited references for background information [32–36].

Some side effects, though not necessarily more common in young adults, are more salient to this group. Appearance, athleticism, sexual potency, autonomy, and self-control are generally highly prized by young adults. Weight gain can occur with many psychotropic medications, especially antipsychotics but also antidepressants and many mood stabilizers. With recognition of body-image concerns in young adults, a clinician may preferentially choose weight-neutral medications, such as lamotrigine, carbamazepine, or bupropion. Sexual side effects, including impotence and delayed/absent orgasm, occur frequently with selective serotonin reuptake inhibitors (SSRIs) and serotonin and norepinephrine reuptake inhibitors (SNRIs). A switch to another drug class or addition of medication to combat the adverse symptoms may be required. Medications for bipolar disorder that cause cognitive slowing and sedation can be a "deal-breaker" for many young adults – especially college students. Discussion of various mood stabilizing strategies, and consideration of the risks and benefits of each option, are necessary. One study using a neurocognitive battery found the following rank order for cognitive impairment for six mood stabilizers, from least to most impairing: lamotrigine, oxcarbazepine, lithium, topiramate, valproate, and carbamazepine [37]. In another study, college athletes with bipolar disorder preferred valproate over lithium, claiming superiority for the former drug in the areas of weight gain, sedation, tremor, and stability of blood levels with dehydration [38].

Some young adults may not have the full executive functioning to weigh the risks and benefits of medication, and to say "Yes, I hate medication. . . but I also do not like being psychotic." Long-term medication adherence is a problem in young adults, who may be tempted to discontinue medication once they are "better," either out of frank denial of the illness or simply from a narcissistic sense of invulnerability to relapse. Consequently, some young adult patients find themselves involved in "revolving door" readmissions to the hospital until they mature enough to interrupt this pattern. These patients may also lack the maturity to engage in frank discussions about illness and to negotiate their concerns about treatment with the clinical team. When, despite best efforts, the patient remains "unconvinced" – as can occur with schizophrenia or mania – the clinician may have to resort to court-ordered medication treatment if the situation warrants.

What issues arise when college students are hospitalized on the inpatient psychiatric unit?

Many young adults admitted to the psychiatric unit are attending college at the time. It is clinically useful to anticipate the issues specific to this population. For instance, students with an extended stay on the unit may be worried about their college courses and grades, or whether they could lose their financial aid [39–41]. There are no universal rules for addressing these issues, since every institution is different. But it is helpful if the patient allows unit staff to contact university officials, who are increasingly astute about mental illness and who generally are interested in maintaining the students in school despite it. When clinical status allows, staff should encourage students to work with the school to plot a course of action with regard to missed classes and examinations, remaining coursework for the semester, and future goals. It is important to realize that the patient may have been unable to perform effectively in school for a period of time leading up to the admission to the hospital, in addition to assignments and deadlines missed during the inpatient stay. In cases where a patient does *not* allow contact with the school, providers may have to work to convince the patient to accept the school's involvement. This negotiation is similar to what occurs when the patient does not allow involvement of his or her family members despite strong recommendations from the team to do so. Finally, since these young adults are in many ways less independent than peers not enrolled in school, in many cases the parents will request or even insist upon input into the care of their children, regardless of the patient's chronological age.

Toward the end of their hospital stay, some college students find that they have remaining symptoms that impair their ability to do well in school. With inpatient lengths of stay becoming shorter and shorter, it is common for patients to require an additional period of recuperation following inpatient treatment for psychotic states, severe depression, and mania. In these cases, a leave of absence from college or a reduced academic load should be considered. For college-aged patients with minimal residual symptoms, a successful return to school will enhance self-esteem and be therapeutic, similar to the return to work for general adult psychiatric patients. Helping college-age patients decide whether or not to return to the family home, versus dormitory room or apartment, after discharge involves looking at a number of variables, including the stability and family dynamics of the home situation, how much of a narcissistic blow it will be to give up the autonomy of living independently, how much support and monitoring the patient will need, and the location of the best resources for ongoing treatment. The unit social worker can help the family and patient sort out these complicated questions as part of discharge planning.

What are the legal issues associated with the treatment of young adults on the unit?

The legal issues that arise with young adult psychiatric inpatients are basically no different than those of adults in general, but a few areas of concern may be more common in this population. For instance, questions related to confidentiality and the duty to safeguard patient disclosures come up frequently with young adult patients. By virtue of their age, from a medicolegal standpoint, young adults have the right to decline family involvement in their treatment, even though they may be acting against their own self-interest in the process. While aligning with the young adult's wish to remain autonomous, the clinician can also work with the patient to sort out the difference between being dependent on one's parents and allowing parents to be helpful. Breaching confidentially may be absolutely necessary when there is a question of the patient's dangerousness toward self or others; clinicians need to know the laws in their jurisdiction, including what situations allow disclosures or create a duty to break confidentiality. The hospital attorney can be helpful with these difficult decisions.

Although statutes may vary from state to state in the United States, young adults with severe mental illnesses can be detained involuntarily in the hospital under certain conditions [42]. Because young adulthood is often the period of onset for schizophrenia and bipolar disorder, it is not uncommon to see young adult patients with major psychiatric illnesses involved in commitment proceedings while on the inpatient unit. There has been increasing attention to a group of patients termed "young adult chronics" [43], who not only end up hospitalized on the inpatient unit, but who are also suitable candidates for legal orders that mandate long-acting antipsychotic medication injections as an outpatient.

What are the pros and cons of mixing young adult patients with older patients?

As long as their specific needs are met, younger adults do well on a psychiatric unit of heterogeneous adult age groups. Although there are some intermediate and long-term programs designed specifically for young adults with psychiatric disorders, many hospitals do not have the number of psychiatric beds that allows separate units for the various age groupings. A cross-generational presence on a psychiatric unit can have certain advantages. Older patients can serve as surrogate parental (or grandparental) figures who can help temper the younger patients' tendencies to act out. Mature middle-aged patients can serve as role models (if stable themselves) of co-operation with treatment.

A homogeneously comprised therapy group that focuses on young adult issues is a welcome addition to unit programming. Any unit that treats young adults should also have the capacity for physical activities, including daily exercise. Young adults also benefit from occupational therapy, recreational therapies, music therapy, and art therapy, each of which usually has enough flexibility to adapt to the needs of the young adult. Especially when group leaders are up to date with current common problems faced by members of the young adult cohort – and maybe even current pop-culture – these groups serve a central function in the day-to-day observation and psychiatric rehabilitation of the young adults on the inpatient unit [13].

What about evaluation and management of suicide risk in young adults?

Suicidal ideation, plans, and actions are implicated in many of the psychiatric hospitalizations of young adults. Suicide itself remains a significant public health issue for young adults in the United States, ranking as the third leading cause of death between the ages of 15 and 24 [44]. With the glut of handguns and other firearms in our country, it is not surprising that firearm injury is the leading cause of death in suicide in this age group, with hanging/suffocation

Table 8.3 Specific risk factors for suicide in hospitalized young adults

Static (non-changing) risk factors:

Personal history of suicidal threats, actions, or self-mutilation

Family history of completed suicides or of major psychiatric illness

History of sexual or physical abuse

Potentially mutable/treatable risk factors:

Current psychiatric illness, negative evaluation of health status

Current symptom picture (anhedonia, hopelessness/helplessness, severe anxiety/panic, chronic pain, command hallucinations)

Intolerable feelings of being alone

Marked identity confusion, including gender/sexual orientation

Acute precipitants to hospitalization (incidents leading to feelings of loss, abandonment, despair, shame, loss of self-esteem, humiliation)

Access to means to harm self, especially firearms

Disruption in relationship with family

Highly formulated suicide plan

Poor treatment alliance with staff and/or failure to accept illness/treatment

and drug overdose/poisoning as the second and third most common methods [45]. An essential part of the evaluation and management of the young adult inpatient therefore involves detailed questioning about the availability of various means of self-harm and special attention to the removal of any firearms from the home prior to the patient's discharge.

The general assessment of suicide is discussed at length elsewhere in this manual (see Chapter 2). But there are some concerns that occur frequently in the assessment and management of suicide risk in the young adult population (Table 8.3). Young adults are particularly sensitive to feelings of failure, loss, and abandonment. It is common to see them admitted to the hospital with suicidal ideation or suicide attempts after a failed romantic relationship, poor academic performance, or a falling out with parents. Young adults struggling with sexual identity are also at heightened risk for suicidality [40], but may be reluctant to disclose this conflict to the inpatient staff. From the standpoint of social supports, risk of suicide in young adults is also heightened by their being in an "in-between stage" – separating from their childhood nuclear family without having a fully formed replacement to buffer life crises. In assessing risk, clinicians should keep in mind that while demographic and diagnostic variables serve as markers of the suicide risk of an individual young adult, the clinician also needs to tune in to the young adult's internal world to determine the particular dynamic that is leading to the wish to die. In other words, it is not enough to determine the Axis I diagnosis and the indicated pharmacologic and/or psychotherapeutic treatment; it is also necessary to determine what problem the young adult patient is trying to solve by suicide. Young adults demonstrate a distinct association between suicidal actions and a constellation of hopelessness, repression, negative life events, impaired interpersonal problem solving, and the inability to recall autobiographical events in specific detail [46]. In light of this finding, the authors of one study suggest that treatment include efforts at enhancing retrieval and integration of memories, a task for which psychotherapy has shown the most success. This process may need to be initiated on the inpatient unit for selected patients, and careful referral to expert outpatient care is crucial.

Members of the inpatient treatment team frequently react negatively to young adult patients admitted to the unit with depression and multiple non-lethal suicide attempts, especially if there is suspicion or history of an Axis II disorder. Since young adults in this group usually also have the physical where-withal to act on their impulses, they are at risk to engage in suicidal or para-suicidal acts on the unit itself, which only serves to increase staff anxiety and sometimes frustration with the patient. And while staff may perceive self-harm or parasuicidal behavior as manipulative and self-absorbed, as a group these patients have considerable psychiatric morbidity – with associated mood, anxiety, and substance use disorders – putting them at high risk for completed suicide at some point. In the inpatient setting, addressing suicide risk in these young adults will entail paying close attention to co-morbid Axis I anxiety disorders, especially including post-traumatic stress disorder (PTSD) and panic disorder; use of substances; and deficits in interpersonal problem-solving and emotional regulation skills.

Which young adult patients are at risk for violence on the inpatient unit?

Because of the relationship between externally directed and internally directed (i.e., suicidal) violent actions, many of the risk factors for violence on the inpatient unit are similar to those for suicide. Despite some media portrayals, schizophrenia in and of itself does not predispose to violence, but command hallucinations or the presence of substance use do increase the risk in this population. Across all young adult patients, substance use, outside of alcohol, is a substantial risk factor for violence, and patients with this history should be approached carefully. Clinicians should be particularly wary of patients with either a history of violence or a diagnosis of antisocial personality disorder [47, 48]. Manic patients can become violent if they feel thwarted or confined, so involuntary status is a violence risk factor especially for this group, but also for inpatients in general.

References

1. Arnett J. Emerging adulthood: a theory of development from the late teens through the twenties. *American Psychologist*, **55**:5 (2000), 469–80.

2. Gogtay N, Giedd J, Lusk L *et al.* Dynamic mapping of human cortical development during childhood through early adulthood. *Proceedings of the National Academy of Sciences*, **101**:21 (2004), 8174.

3. Pujol J, Vendrell P, Junqué C, Martí-Vilalta J & Capdevila A. When does human brain development end? Evidence of corpus callosum growth up to adulthood. *Annals of Neurology*, **34**:1 (1993), 71–5.

4. Sowell E R, Thompson P M, Holmes C J, Jernigan T L & Toga A W. In vivo evidence for post-adolescent brain maturation in frontal and striatal regions. *Nature Neuroscience*, **2**:10 (1999), 859–61.

5. Erikson E. *Childhood and Society*. New York: W.W. Norton & Co., Inc.; 1950.

6. Ford E, Rosenberg M, Holsten M & Boudreaux T. Managing sexual behavior on adult acute care inpatient psychiatric units. *Psychiatric Services*, **54**:3 (2003), 346–50.

7. Ticho G R. Female autonomy and young adult women. *Journal of the American Psychoanalytic Association*, **24**:5 Suppl (1976), 139–55.

8. Blos P. *On Adolescence: A Psychoanalytic Interpretation*. New York: Free Press of Glencoe; 1962.

9. Blos P. *The Adolescent Passage: Developmental Issues*. New York: International Universities Press; 1979.

10. Colarusso C. Separation–individuation phenomena in adulthood: general concepts and the fifth individuation. *Journal of the American Psychoanalytic Association*, **48**:4 (2000), 1467–89.

11. Winnicott D W. *The Maturational Processes and the Facilitating Environment: Studies in the Theory of Emotional Development*. London: Hogarth Press; 1965.

12. Glangeaud-Freudenthal N & Barnett B. Mother–baby inpatient psychiatric care in different countries: data collection and issues – Introduction. *Archives of Women's Mental Health*, **7**:1 (2004), 49–51.

13. Snyder S. Comprehensive inpatient treatment for the young adult patient. *Psychiatric Hospital*, **15**:3 (1984), 119–25.

14. Winnicott D W. Transitional objects and transitional phenomena: a study of the first not-me possession. *International Journal of Psycho-Analysis*, **34**:2 (1953), 89–97.

15. Cardasis W, Hochman J A & Silk K R. Transitional objects and borderline personality disorder. *American Journal of Psychiatry*, **154**:2 (1997), 250–5.

16. Tohen M, Bromet E, Murphy J & Tsuang M. Psychiatric epidemiology. *Harvard Review of Psychiatry*, **8**:3 (2000), 111–25.

17. Kessler R, Berglund P, Demler O *et al.* Lifetime prevalence and age-of-onset distributions of DSM-IV disorders in the National Comorbidity Survey Replication. *Archives of General Psychiatry*, **62**:6 (2005), 593.

18. Lewinsohn P, Seeley J, Buckley M & Klein D. Bipolar disorder in adolescence and young adulthood. *Child and Adolescent Psychiatric Clinics of North America*, **11**:3 (2002), 461–75.

19. Deans C & Meocevic E. Attitudes of registered psychiatric nurses towards patients diagnosed with borderline personality disorder. *Contemporary Nurse*, **21**:1 (2006), 43–9.

20. Rossberg J, Karterud S, Pedersen G & Friis S. An empirical study of countertransference reactions toward patients with personality disorders. *Comprehensive Psychiatry*, **48**:3 (2007), 225–230.

21. Zanarini M C, Frankenburg F R, Hennen J, Reich D B & Silk K R. Prediction of the 10-year course of borderline personality disorder. *American Journal of Psychiatry*, **163**:5 (2006), 827–32.

22. Carpenter W T Jr. Evidence-based treatment for first-episode schizophrenia? *American Journal of Psychiatry*, **158**:11 (2001), 1771–3.

23. Harrow M, Sands J R, Silverstein M L & Goldberg J F. Course and outcome for schizophrenia versus other psychotic patients: a longitudinal study. *Schizophrenia Bulletin*, **23**:2 (1997), 287–303.

24. Jobe T H & Harrow M. Long-term outcome of patients with schizophrenia: a review. *Canadian Journal of Psychiatry*, **50**:14 (2005), 892–900.

25. Christie K A, Burke J D Jr, Regier D A *et al.* Epidemiologic evidence for early onset of mental disorders and higher risk of drug abuse in young adults. *American Journal of Psychiatry*, **145**:8 (1988), 971–5.

26. Weitzman E R S M. Poor mental health, depression, and associations with alcohol consumption, harm, and abuse in a national sample of young adults in college. *Journal of Nervous & Mental Disease*, **192**:4 (2004), 269–77.

27. Miller W R & Rollnick S. *Motivational Interviewing: Preparing People for Change*, 2nd edn. New York: Guilford Press; 2002.

28. Casey D. Clozapine: neuroleptic-induced EPS and tardive dyskinesia. *Psychopharmacology*, **99** (1989), 47–53.

29. Moller H-J, Baldwin D S, Goodwin G *et al.* Do SSRIs or antidepressants in general increase suicidality? WPA Section on Pharmacopsychiatry: consensus statement. *European Archives of Psychiatry & Clinical Neuroscience*, **258**:Suppl. 3 (2008), 3–23.

30. Gunnell D, Saperia J & Ashby D. Selective serotonin reuptake inhibitors (SSRIs) and suicide in adults: meta-analysis of drug company data from placebo controlled, randomised controlled trials submitted to the MHRA's safety review. *British Medical Journal*, **330**:7488 (2005), 385.

31. Simon G, Savarino J, Operskalski B & Wang P. Suicide risk during antidepressant treatment. *American Journal of Psychiatry*, **163**:1 (2006), 41.

32. Alwan S, Reefhuis J, Rasmussen S, Olney R & Friedman J. Use of selective serotonin-reuptake inhibitors in pregnancy and the risk of birth defects. *New England Journal of Medicine*, **356**:26 (2007), 2684.

33. Cohen L, Altshuler L, Harlow B *et al.* Relapse of major depression during pregnancy in women who maintain or discontinue antidepressant treatment. *Journal of the American Medical Association*, **295**:5 (2006), 499.

34. Lin H, Chen I, Chen Y, Lee H & Wu F. Maternal schizophrenia and pregnancy outcome: does the use of antipsychotics make a difference? *Schizophrenia Research*, **116**:1 (2010), 55–60.

35. Weissman A, Levy B, Hartz A *et al.* Pooled analysis of antidepressant levels in lactating mothers, breast milk, and nursing infants. *American Journal of Psychiatry*, **161**:6 (2004), 1066.

36. Yonkers K, Wisner K, Stowe Z *et al.* Management of bipolar disorder during pregnancy and the postpartum period. *American Journal of Psychiatry*, **161**:4 (2004), 608.

37. Gualtieri C T & Johnson L G. Comparative neurocognitive effects of 5 psychotropic anticonvulsants and lithium. *Medscape General Medicine*, **8**:3 (2006).

38. Broshek D K & Freeman J R. Psychiatric and neuropsychological issues in sport medicine. *Clinics in Sports Medicine*, **24**:3 (2005), 663–79.

39. Kessler R, Foster C, Saunders W & Stang P. Social consequences of psychiatric disorders. I: Educational attainment. *American Journal of Psychiatry*, **152**:7 (1995), 1026.

40. Eisenberg D, Gollust S E, Golberstein E & Hefner J L. Prevalence and correlates of depression, anxiety, and suicidality among university students. *American Journal of Orthopsychiatry*, **77**:4 (2007), 534–42.

41. Megivern D, Pellerito S & Mowbray C. Barriers to higher education for individuals with psychiatric disabilities. *Psychiatric Rehabilitation Journal*, **26**:3 (2003), 217–31.

42. Treatment Advocacy Center. State Standards for Assisted Treatment: State by State Chart. September 2008; www.treatmentadvocacycenter.org [Accessed September 23, 2009].

43. Cournos F & Melle S L. The young adult chronic patient: a look back. *Psychiatric Services*, **51**:8 (2000), 996–1000.

44. National Vital Statistics Reports http://www.cdc.gov/nch/data/nvsr57/nvsr57 [Accessed April 17, 2009].

45. CDC. Centers for Disease Control and Prevention http://www.cdc.gov/injury/wisqars/index.html.

46. Arie M, Apter A, Orbach I, Yefet Y & Zalzman G. Autobiographical memory, interpersonal problem solving, and suicidal behavior in adolescent inpatients. *Comprehensive Psychiatry*, **49**:1 (2008), 22–9.

47. Soliman AE-D & Reza H. Risk factors and correlates of violence among acutely ill adult psychiatric inpatients. *Psychiatric Services*, **52**:1 (2001), 75–80.

48. Zhang J, McKeown R E, Hussey J R, Thompson S J & Woods J R. Gender differences in risk factors for attempted suicide among young adults: findings from the Third National Health and Nutrition Examination Survey. *Annals of Epidemiology*, **15**:2 (2005), 167–174.

Clinical documentation on the inpatient unit

When specific diagnoses are mentioned, we are referring to diagnoses and criteria as listed in the *Diagnostic and Statistical Manual of Mental Disorders*, 4th edition, text revision (DSM-IV-TR) unless otherwise specified.

Who reads clinical notes?

The potentially *large* audience for clinical documentation can be divided into smaller groups across several domains (Figure 9.1). Considering the question of *who* – potential readers are clinicians, overseers, and patients [1, 2]. Patients as readers are addressed separately below. (Of course, one must also consider attorneys, judges, juries, and expert witnesses; but the medicolegal perspective is also considered separately below.) The group of clinicians includes oneself, other team members, trainees, consulting colleagues, and the patient's future providers. Overseers can include internal utilization review (UR) staff, individuals performing external UR (i.e., on behalf of third-party payers), internal quality assurance (QA) assessors, and external QA assessors (i.e., regulators and licensing agencies) [3–6].

Why do all of these people read the medical record?

The *why* question is answered easily for the clinician group. For these people, notes are all about the care of the patient. For the provider writing the note, it is often literally "taking notes" for him/herself on the patient's problems, the treatment plan, and the day-to-day progress. The chart is also the primary mode of information transfer among members of the treatment team, though of course it can not replace real-time verbal communication. In the modern psychiatric unit, high turnover and hectic pace are often at odds with the need for an authentic interdisciplinary approach. Effective documentation can make all of the pertinent information available to all of the team members no matter when or where they need it. Finally, the medical record is the "final repository of information on the patient's illness and treatment" [3].

Future providers, whether just collecting a medical history or assuming primary responsibility for the care of the patient in the hospital or clinic, will

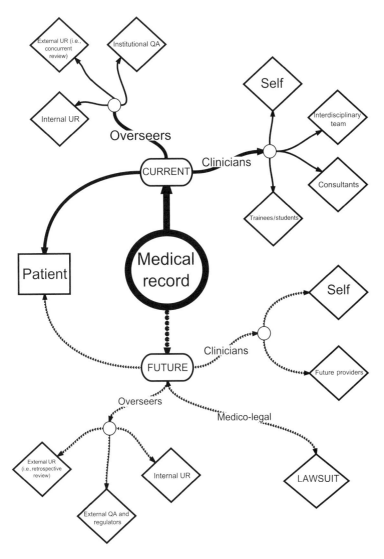

Figure 9.1 Who reads the medical record?

rely on this one source for information regarding months, years, even decades of treatment of the patient's illness. The quality of previous clinical documentation for a new patient can be a wonderful boost or a terrible hindrance to the new clinician's ability to provide effective, efficient care.

On the other hand, addressing the *why* question for the overseers group is much more complex, and mostly beyond the scope of this volume. The inpatient clinician "serves many masters." Both during and after a patient's hospitalization, there will likely be several people asking questions about the patient's care, most of the time via the medical record.

Most institutions have a UR staff that is tasked with the responsibility of making sure the institutional criteria for admission and/or continued stay are met. These people often are also the conduit of clinical information from the inpatient unit to the external reviewers. Regardless of whether a region has universal health care or not, someone is still paying the bill. Therefore, there is always some level of external review to make sure that resources are being used appropriately. In the United States, this often means regular communication with the patient's insurance company, during the process of "concurrent review." The intensity of the scrutiny depends on the patient's specific policy and the contract that the institution has with the payer. Even in cases where concurrent review is not performed, e.g., with Medicare or some "traditional" insurance plans, "retrospective review" is still employed to check up on providers and institutions.

Every jurisdiction or government body has policies and procedures regarding licensing, accreditation, and quality assurance. Institutions, individual units, and individual providers are responsible for operating within the guidelines that are set forth by several different levels of regulators. Non-compliance with these policies can result in a fine or other probationary action, or in serious cases even suspension of license or unit closure. The groups that make these decisions rely on information gathered from surveys, site visits, and, yes, the medical records of patients treated in the facility.

What are the essential functions of clinical notes in inpatient psychiatry?

Another way to examine clinical documentation in psychiatry is consideration of *what* the notes are supposed to accomplish. It is still useful to organize the list according to the various readers (Table 9.1). Again, medicolegal situations are discussed in more detail further on.

Among the readers listed in Table 9.1, reviewers for insurance companies and anyone associated with potential legal action incite the most anxiety in professionals who complete clinical documentation. In the United States, reimbursement for psychiatric care is lower than for almost any other service, and inpatient days are often approved only a few at a time – especially by managed care organizations [4, 5]. Therefore, sometimes the inpatient progress note turns into a daily plea for a little bit more time to help the patient. This situation

Table 9.1 Essential functions of clinical notes

Oneself	reminders of past encounters with the patient
	running problem list, "to-do" list
Other team members	integration of various parts of patient's care
	information about patient through time and across settings
	education of trainees (e.g., case conferences)
Colleagues	summary of the course so far to bring one's replacement up to speed
	summary of the course so far to provide background to a consultant
Utilization reviewers	evidence that the patient meets clinical standards for level of care
	ongoing demonstration of appropriate care, competent provider
Regulators, QA staff	review of bad outcomes to improve methods, procedures
	evidence of adherence to guidelines and policies
Participants in legal proceeding	evidence that standards of care were/were not met
	evidence for/against negligence
	evidence that provider is/is not competent

can lead to excessive focus on proving one's case in the clinical note, and often can lead to excessive length of the notes as well [6]. That said, following the advice in Fauman's volume [3], even though it is focused on documenting in a managed-care environment, will lead a clinician to cover most, perhaps all, of what the other readers are looking for as well. As listed on page 92, notes should answer the following four questions: Why does the patient need the level of care you are requesting now? What are you trying to accomplish with the care and how will you know when you have accomplished it? How will you treat the patient? What are you planning to do with the patient after discharge? [3].

What are the characteristics of good clinical notes?

Numerous adjectives can be applied to distinguish "good" from "bad" notes [7]. Narrowing the list as much as possible, one ends up with "clear," "concise," and "complete" [2, 8, 9]. Even though a clinician's notes have a diverse audience, each member of which likely has a different set of expectations, this relatively simple advice is still sufficient as a guiding principle for clinical documentation. The clinical note is really just a collection of data.

As long as the various interested parties are able to find the information they need easily and efficiently, then the writer of the note really can please everyone.

Clarity *should* be the easiest of the three to achieve. But anyone who has examined records from even just a handful of different providers knows that this characteristic is not universal. Although many providers are now employing electronic medical records (EMRs), many still are not [10]. And even among EMR users, very few institutions are truly "paperless." Handwriting legibility is still a major problem, especially when compounded by the poor resolution of fax machines [6, 11]. If parts of the clinical documentation are handwritten, the provider must write legibly. Even in the electronic world, clarity is not a given. The overuse of copy–paste functions in electronic notes can render them useless in terms of displaying useful information [6, 12]. Electronic medical records are discussed more below.

Conciseness is one of the most challenging lessons to learn in any kind of clinical training and one of the most challenging lessons for supervisors to teach [13]. It is the mark of wisdom and experience to convey, with just a few carefully chosen words, information that meets all of the goals outlined above. Joseph M. Williams, in an early edition of his popular style manual, said it best: "...you can usually be more concise and direct if you simply present the most salient observations and conclusions, minus the metadiscourse or narrative" [14]. Put more simply: "Say what you mean – no more, no less."

Completeness is the most studied quality factor in the growing field of clinical informatics [7]. Missing information in a patient's chart is not only frustrating for a reviewing clinician, but can also be dangerous for the patient [11]. What makes a note complete is different for each type of note (see below) and must take into account all of the functions of notes discussed so far. A popular mantra in the medical malpractice world is "if it isn't documented, it wasn't done" [2]. This idea applies more broadly of course. An institution will not be reimbursed for care provided unless the details are documented. A future colleague might try to "reinvent the wheel" if notes in the patient's record do not contain enough information about treatment trials. However, complete does not mean *all*-encompassing. "There will always be questions from reviewers and others. Don't try always to predict what the questions are going to be" [1]. If a provider spends all of her/his time predicting what people might be looking for in the chart in the future, no time will be left for patient care.

What are the basic types of clinical notes on the inpatient psychiatric unit?

There are three basic types of clinical notes on the inpatient psychiatric unit: admission note, progress note, and discharge summary. They may be called something else: specific institutional practices vary. Also, individual members

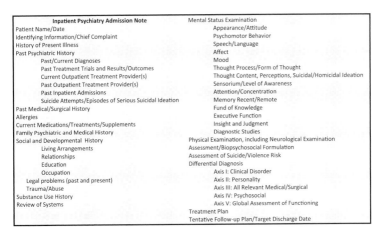

Inpatient Psychiatry Admission Note	Mental Status Examination
Patient Name/Date	Appearance/Attitude
Identifying Information/Chief Complaint	Psychomotor Behavior
History of Present Illness	Speech/Language
Past Psychiatric History	Affect
Past/Current Diagnoses	Mood
Past Treatment Trials and Results/Outcomes	Thought Process/Form of Thought
Current Outpatient Treatment Provider(s)	Thought Content, Perceptions, Suicidal/Homicidal Ideation
Past Outpatient Treatment Provider(s)	Sensorium/Level of Awareness
Past Inpatient Admissions	Attention/Concentration
Suicide Attempts/Episodes of Serious Suicidal Ideation	Memory Recent/Remote
Past Medical/Surgical History	Fund of Knowledge
Allergies	Executive Function
Current Medications/Treatments/Supplements	Insight and Judgment
Family Psychiatric and Medical History	Diagnostic Studies
Social and Developmental History	Physical Examination, including Neurological Examination
Living Arrangements	Assessment/Biopsychosocial Formulation
Relationships	Assessment of Suicide/Violence Risk
Education	Differential Diagnosis
Occupation	Axis I: Clinical Disorder
Legal problems (past and present)	Axis II: Personality
Trauma/Abuse	Axis III: All Relevant Medical/Surgical
Substance Use History	Axis IV: Psychosocial
Review of Systems	Axis V: Global Assessment of Functioning
	Treatment Plan
	Tentative Follow-up Plan/Target Discharge Date

Figure 9.2 Admission note template.

of the multidisciplinary team may document their own versions of each of these; but the general idea is the same everywhere. On admission, providers must gather all of the information that explains why the patient is being admitted and what the initial assessment and plan are. At some interval, usually daily, the team must document updates to the patient's status and explain changes in that assessment and plan. Finally, there is a single document that serves to summarize the entire treatment course, which is often sent to the patient's outpatient provider(s) as well [17, 18].

The admission note serves to address the following:

Why is the patient here?

What does the team think the problems are?

How does the team plan to address each problem?

What are the expected results of the interventions?

What is the plan for when the patient leaves the hospital?

Depending on the policies of the institution and the complexity of the case, this document could be one page or ten pages. Figure 9.2 shows an example template that can be used for an admission note.

Progress notes are the running commentary of inpatient psychiatry. Patients are admitted to psychiatric units because they need close observation, support, and treatment. Interval progress notes are the legal record of those aspects of a patient's care. These documents address:

```
Inpatient Psychiatry Progress Note
Patient Name/Date
Contact and Coordination Time
Interval History
Mental Status Examination
Vital Signs/Physical Assessment
Laboratory Results
Other Studies
Current Medications
Assessment
Suicide/Violence Risk Assessment
Differential Diagnosis
General medical/surgical problems
Justification for Continued Hospitalization
Plan
Target Discharge Date
```

Figure 9.3 Progress note template.

What happened since the last note?

What key observations have team members made?

What is the status of the patient's current problems?

Are there any new problems?

Have there been any complications?

What adjustments to the plan are necessary and what are the expected results?

What is the plan for when the patient leaves the hospital?

Figure 9.3 shows an example inpatient progress note template.

Finally, the discharge summary is an organized presentation of all of the relevant data from the patient's hospital stay. This is often the only document that a patient's primary medical and mental health providers have access to, unless his/her outpatient care is in the same "system" as the inpatient unit. The discharge summary should include a description of the patient's status on admission; major decisions, events, and interventions during the inpatient stay; and the patient's status on the day of discharge. This document should also list the patient's final diagnoses (which may differ from those on admission), an updated medication list, and specific recommendations for follow up including scheduled appointments and reasons that the patient should return to the hospital or emergency department. A "Hospital course" section should address the following:

What was the patient's demeanor in the hospital?

To what extent did the patient actively participate in treatment?

What medication changes were carried out and what were the results?

What psychological interventions were employed and what were the results?

Figure 9.4 Discharge summary template.

Inpatient Psychiatry Discharge Summary
Patient Name
Admission Date
Discharge Date
Inpatient Provider(s)
Principal Diagnoses
Secondary Diagnoses/Chronic Medical Problems
Pertinent Labs, Procedures, and Studies
Final Discharge Medications
Allergies
Clinical Course
Brief Summary of Admission HPI
Admission Mental Status Examination
Hospital Course
Discharge Status
Discharge Mental Status Examination
Current Assessment/Biopsychosocial Formulation
Current Suicide/Violence Risk Assessment
Unresolved Issues
Recommended Follow-up/Scheduled Appointments
Instructions for returning to ED or hospital

How were social issues handled? (e.g., family meeting(s), applications for government aid)

Were there any complications or adverse events, and how were they addressed?

Figure 9.4 shows an example discharge summary template.

What *is* an assessment (a.k.a "formulation," a.k.a. "impression")?

The assessment is the meat of the clinical document. It is the *only* part of the whole process of caring for a patient that only a trained practitioner can contribute. The assessment integrates the patient's history, collateral information, the team's observations, and the "hard data" provided by the laboratory and/or radiology department. The collation of this sometimes huge volume of information into "a few pithy sentences that describe diagnosis and plan and what you expect to see" [1] is a skill that is the frustration of trainees and the trademark of experience and wisdom. This assessment will also evolve throughout the hospital stay with accumulation of data and deepening understanding of the patient, to the point where the final assessment in the

Table 9.2 *In our experience*. . . Hints for a good "assessment" after the initial evaluation

Do not insert new historical information in the assessment; it should only pull together elements of the preceding sections of the evaluation.

The assessment section can allow for speculation about differential diagnosis.

Point out the likely stressors that led to the hospitalization, which will give you a treatment focus for psychosocial interventions.

Do not neglect the role of biological factors including medical illness, history of head injury, genetic loading, substance use, and/or poor compliance with medications.

Psychological factors can be phrased in terms of cognitive distortions, defects in coping strategies, core conflicts and maladaptive defense mechanisms, injuries to self-esteem, and/or reactions to grief and loss.

Think about the reader. Try to be concise. Avoid too much technical jargon.

Remember: The assessment is basically what you think is "going on" with the patient.

discharge summary is less tentative and more refined than that of the initial evaluation.

Many training programs teach the usefulness of the biopsychosocial model [15, 16]. Though not without its detractors [17], at the very least it is a reminder of all of the various factors involved when a patient is ill enough to warrant admission to the inpatient psychiatric unit. As mentioned previously in this manual, it is not the diagnosis alone that brings a patient into the hospital, but the interactions between the illness and life events, relationships, expectations, and circumstances. "Psychosocial factors may operate to facilitate, sustain or modify the course of illness, even though their relative weight may vary from illness to illness, from one individual to another and even between two different episodes of the same illness in the same individual" [18]. (See Table 9.2.)

What is the role of clinical documentation in malpractice defense?

This topic is addressed separately not because it is necessarily the most important, but because it is the most likely to provoke anxiety among clinicians practicing in any potentially litigious setting. Looking at the big picture, it is difficult to identify parts of clinical notes that *only* serve to "tell it to the jury *before* you get sued." Adherence to the guidelines presented in this chapter should result in notes that also protect one in court. A general principle is that good clinical documentation is going to support your case, if it even gets that far. If the clinician has maintained good clinical documentation, there may not even be a lawsuit because potential plaintiff's attorneys will see a very difficult case ahead [11, 19].

Good documentation performs two major roles if a malpractice suit does proceed to trial. First, the medical record is the legal document that describes the events of the case [2, 9]. It is "the witness who never loses his memory" [1]. More generally, and perhaps more importantly, the quality of the medical documentation paints a general picture of the defendant's credibility. Charting that is clear, concise, and complete paints the picture of a practitioner who is conscientious, caring, and competent. This is the main reason that poor documentation is a "kiss of death" in the legal arena [11].

Documentation in the context of malpractice defense is a complex issue, with myriad factors that must be considered. The article by Soisson *et al.* [20], though somewhat dated and focused on psychotherapists, addresses most of the issues still plaguing clinicians today. Weaver's bulletin [2], written for emergency medicine providers, is a great reference for more current policies and requirements.

How important is documentation of suicide assessments and related decisions?

It is extremely important to document, in detail, all findings of one's comprehensive suicide assessment [19]. It is important to remember the old adage mentioned above, "if it isn't documented, it wasn't done" [2]. Psychiatrists are not perfect prognosticators when it comes to suicide risk, and even a state-of-the-art assessment and prolonged hospitalization cannot prevent all occurrences of suicidal acts. Forensic psychiatrists tell us that courts want to see that the clinician practiced a reasonable standard of care in assessing and treating suicidal patients [20, 21]. The clinician should document his or her thought process and the associated risk/benefit analysis that leads to specific decisions, such as allowing the patient to leave on pass or the changing observation level. This level of detail is necessary even if there are no "abnormalities" or "significant issues" [2].

Furthermore, the chart is a method of communication between providers. On the busy inpatient service, sometimes a new clinician is assuming responsibility for the care of a patient on the patient's planned day of discharge. The provider rotating off must leave a carefully documented, complete risk assessment in the chart, and ideally communicate it directly to his/her colleague as well. Otherwise the new provider must do one of the following: (1) perform a brand-new, comprehensive risk assessment, instead of a focused, follow-up interview, before discharge; (2) discharge the patient based only on the report that "this is the discharge day;" or (3) keep the patient an extra day or more to "get to know" the patient him-/herself. In this day of managed care, utilization review, and extreme demands on clinicians' (especially physicians') time, none of the above is acceptable.

Are there things that should *not* be documented in the chart?

Much of the clinical work on inpatient psychiatric units involves description of the patients' physical presence, interactions with peers and staff, and behavior. Sometimes characteristics in these categories do not fall within the limits of what is deemed "socially acceptable." For example, a psychotic patient with the delusional belief that the city water in her apartment is poisoned might avoid bathing for a long period of time. She will likely be "malodorous" on admission to the hospital. If her ability to care for herself is examined in court during the involuntary commitment process, the patient might find out that she was described as "malodorous." Maybe it would be better to say "needs to improve hygiene" or even "appeared as if she had not bathed in some time" – or maybe not. It is probably best to avoid using pejorative adjectives (e.g., "manipulative" or "whiny") to describe behaviors. Besides often reflecting countertransference attitudes on the part of the clinician, such terms in the written record can undermine the treatment alliance if the patient reads his or her chart, and can be used by a plaintiff's attorney to demonstrate an unsympathetic attitude toward the patient. The point is not to phrase everything in a vague, circuitous way, but to at least consider what the patient's response would be when/if they see their chart [22]. As long as the description is written in such a way that a good clinician reading it knows what he or she needs to know, the record has done its job [1].

> A 74-year-old man has been feeling so depressed recently that he "want[s] God to take [him]." Despite that, he appears and interacts like someone who is euthymic, such as smiling and making overly-polite comments to the clinician. In the mental status examination, the provider records that the patient's affect "is inappropriate to recent history, current circumstances, and stated mood." For the next several months there is a positive treatment alliance, and the patient's depression improves markedly with medication and brief psychotherapy. Then, in preparation for a medical procedure, the patient requests and receives a copy of his psychiatric records. The patient then calls the clinician the following week and "fires" him. The patient's wife sends a message explaining that the patient is upset that he was described as "inappropriate."

Although mental health providers' job is to render opinions and offer treatment, one must be careful about what types of opinions are placed in the medical record. An opinion about a diagnosis or whether a patient can manage his or her own finances is what clinicians are supposed to offer. But the opinion that it is "unfortunate that the patient fell" after starting a medication known to cause orthostatic hypotension is something to avoid. First, it is unnecessary – of course one does not want one's patients to fall. Second, it adds emotional content to the facts regarding a known possible side effect. A plaintiff's attorney could ask, "Doctor, if you thought it was so unfortunate that the patient fell, why did you cause her to do so by prescribing this medication?"

What about tailoring notes to specific purposes or audiences?

Every word that is included or left out of a clinical note represents a choice that the provider makes. Extracting important information from the swirl of data that surrounds each patient is an important part of one's job on the inpatient unit; a major focus of training; and an essential step in achieving the clear, concise, and complete notes described above. This chapter also encourages clinicians to consider the various readers who might encounter the chart in the future. So if the writer of the note is already filtering information and is documenting with the future audience in mind, it might make sense to try to make everyone's life easier by tweaking things just a bit more to make sure the patient gets the best care possible.

> A depressed homeless woman on the inpatient unit is no longer feeling suicidal. Her mood is much improved and she is no longer hopeless about her future. The multidisciplinary team assesses her risk of suicide as low. The psychiatrist knows that the Medicaid reviewer is not going to authorize continuing days of inpatient treatment based on that. But, it is extremely cold outside, and the local shelter will not have an opening until tomorrow. Furthermore, the patient's social worker has developed a strong alliance with her and has convinced her to attend substance treatment. That social worker is at a conference today, but will be back tomorrow with a promised referral to a local treatment program.

It appears that the "easy" way of handling this situation is to keep the patient in the hospital one more day, allowing her to go to the shelter instead of the street, and giving her a more cohesive follow-up plan. But in order to have the additional day paid for, the patient would have to be suicidal. Everyone who suffers from depression, co-morbid substance use, and is homeless is at some risk of suicide. So the psychiatrist documents that the patient continues "to be at risk for suicide" and decides not to write details about her improvement or the team's formal assessment in the progress note for the day.

Dwyer and Shih [23] argue, and the authors agree, that the actions above represent dishonesty on the part of the psychiatrist. It undermines the integrity of the treatment alliance between provider and patient, of the relationship between the psychiatrist and the team, and the social and legal contracts between the psychiatrist and the community. As pointed out in the referenced paper, there are alternatives besides turning the woman out into the cold or lying in the chart – though these alternatives rarely are the "easy" way to address the problem. Speaking with the reviewer from the insurance plan would be one option. Discussing with the patient other people with whom she could stay for one night would be another.

References

1. Fauman M A. Personal communication. Ann Arbor, MI; 2009.

2. Weaver J C. Appropriate documentation: your first (and best) defense. *ED Legal Letter*, May 1, 2004.

3. Fauman M A. *Negotiating Managed Care: A Manual For Clinicians*. American Psychiatric Publishing, Inc.

4. Sharfstein S S & Dickerson F B. Hospital psychiatry for the twenty-first century. *Health Affairs*, **28**:3 (2009), 685–8.

5. Wickizer T M, Lessler D & Travis K M. Controlling inpatient psychiatric utilization through managed care. *American Journal of Psychiatry*, **153**:3 (1996), 339–45.

6. Hartzband P & Groopman J. Off the record: avoiding the pitfalls of going electronic. *New England Journal of Medicine*, **358**:16 (2008), 1656.

7. Stetson P D, Morrison F P, Bakken S & Johnson S B. Preliminary development of the physician documentation quality instrument. *Journal of the American Medical Information Association*, **15**:4 (2008), 534–41.

8. Lyons J & Martinez J. Medical malpractice matters: medical record. *Current Surgery*, **62**:6 (2005), 653–6.

9. Murphy B J. Principles of good medical record documentation. *Journal of Medical Practice Management*, **16**:5 (2001), 258–60.

10. Ford E W, Menachemi N, Peterson L T & Huerta T R. Resistance is futile: but it is slowing the pace of EHR adoption nonetheless. *Journal of the American Medical Information Association*, **16**:3 (2009), 274–81.

11. Kightlinger R. Sloppy records: the kiss of death for a malpractice defense. *Medical Economics*, **76**:11 (1999), 166–74.

12. Hammond K W, Helbig S T, Benson C C & Brathwaite-Sketoe B M. Are electronic medical records trustworthy? Observations on copying, pasting and duplication. *AMIA Annual Symposium Proceedings*, (2003), 269–73.

13. Coakley F, Heinze S, Shadbolt C *et al*. Routine editing of trainee-generated radiology reports effect on style quality. *Academic Radiology*, **10**:3 (2003), 289–94.

14. Williams J M. *Style: Ten Lessons in Clarity and Grace.* Glenview, IL: Scott Foresman; 1981.

15. Engel G L. The need for a new medical model: a challenge for biomedicine. *Science*, **196**:4286 (1977), 129–36.

16. Engel G L. From biomedical to biopsychosocial. Being scientific in the human domain. *Psychosomatics*, **38**:6 (1997), 521–8.

17. McLaren N. Interactive dualism as a partial solution to the mind–brain problem for psychiatry. *Medical Hypotheses*, **66**:6 (2006), 1165–73.

18. Fava G A & Sonino N. The biopsychosocial model thirty years later. *Psychotherapy and Psychosomatics*, **77**:1 (2008), 1–2.

19. Simpson S & Stacy M. Avoiding the malpractice snare: documenting suicide risk assessment. *Journal of Psychiatric Practice*, **10**:3 (2004), 185–9.

20. Soisson E L, VandeCreek L & Knapp S. Thorough record keeping: a good defense in a litigious era. *Professional Psychology: Research and Practice*, **18**:5 (1987), 498–502.

21. Simon R. *Concise Guide to Psychiatry and Law for Clinicians.* Washington: American Psychiatric Press, Inc.; 1992.

22. Wadden T A & Didie E. What's in a name? Patients' preferred terms for describing obesity. *Obesity Research*, **11**:9 (2003), 1140–6.

23. Dwyer J & Shih A. The ethics of tailoring the patient's chart. *Psychiatric Services*, **49**:10 (1998), 1309.

Index